I0414478

THE 18%
SOLUTION

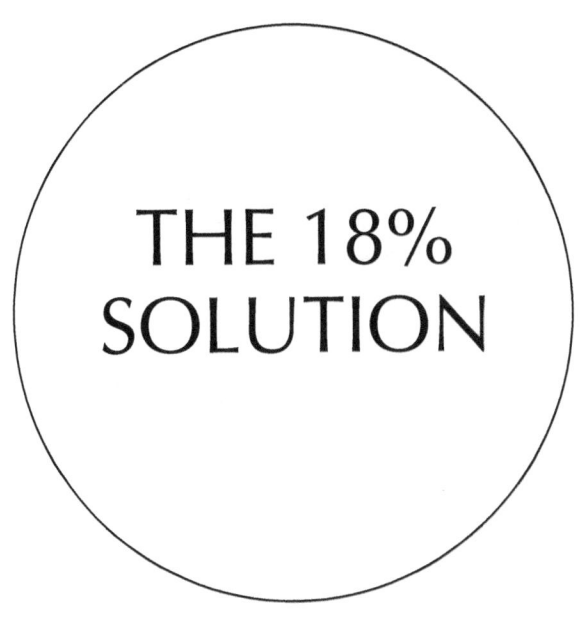

THE 18% SOLUTION

LOSE 18 PERCENT OF YOUR WEIGHT IN 18 WEEKS

HARRY WEISMAN, M.D.

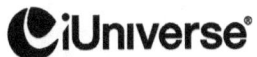

THE 18% SOLUTION
LOSE 18 PERCENT OF YOUR WEIGHT IN 18 WEEKS

Copyright © 2007 Harry Weisman, M.D.

All rights reserved. No part of this book may be used or reproduced by any means, graphic, electronic, or mechanical, including photocopying, recording, taping or by any information storage retrieval system without the written permission of the author except in the case of brief quotations embodied in critical articles and reviews.

iUniverse books may be ordered through booksellers or by contacting:

iUniverse
1663 Liberty Drive
Bloomington, IN 47403
www.iuniverse.com
1-800-Authors (1-800-288-4677)

Because of the dynamic nature of the Internet, any web addresses or links contained in this book may have changed since publication and may no longer be valid. The views expressed in this work are solely those of the author and do not necessarily reflect the views of the publisher, and the publisher hereby disclaims any responsibility for them.

Any people depicted in stock imagery provided by Getty Images are models, and such images are being used for illustrative purposes only.
Certain stock imagery © Getty Images.

ISBN: 978-0-5954-2566-2 (sc)
ISBN: 978-0-5958-6895-7 (e)

Print information available on the last page.

iUniverse rev. date: 04/03/2019

To the memory of my father,
who encouraged me to work towards excellence
And in gratitude toward my mother,
who always encouraged me to become a physician

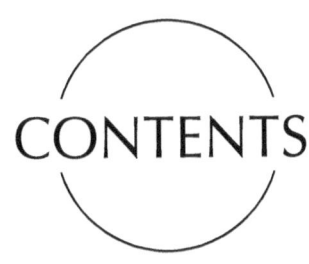

CONTENTS

(Continued)

AUTHOR'S NOTE

A word of thanks to Michael Levin, who helped me put my thoughts down on paper in a logical way.

Thanks also to my many wonderful patients who inspired and encouraged me to write this book. As they lost, we all gained.

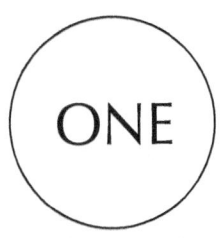

ONE

THE DOCTOR WHO NEEDED TO DIET

I never intended to become a diet doctor. I never even wanted to go on a diet! Nor am I a diet doctor by training. I am an endocrinologist, and an Assistant Clinical Professor of Medicine at UCLA School of Medicine. I've specialized for twenty seven years in treating people with hormone-related medical issues, such as diabetes, thyroid diseases, metabolism issues, and cholesterol disorders.

The only problem was that like many doctors, I had become terribly overweight myself. I'm six foot one inches tall, and I weighed an unhealthy 235 pounds. My weight situation was affecting my stamina, my energy level, and my self-esteem. More to the point, my overweight status was seriously undermining my credibility with my patients. Here I was, sitting in a white doctor's lab coat at my desk at the prestigious UCLA Medical Center, telling people facing diabetes and high cholesterol, among other medical problems, that they needed to lose a lot of weight in order to battle these diseases. And yet I needed to lose a lot of weight—sometimes more than some of my patients!

It began to grate on my conscience that I was telling my patients to do as I said, not as I did. What kind of example was I setting for them? As a trained endocrinologist, I knew better than most lay people, of course, the risks and dangers inherent in carrying too much weight. I knew that I was a likely candidate for many if not all of the illnesses that I treated. On top of that, it just bothered me personally that I weighed so much, that I couldn't jog as quickly or as far as I liked, and that, quite frankly, I was so out of control with regard to food.

There's no doubt about it—I *was* out of control with regard to food. I am an absolute food addict, a foodaholic, and a chronic binger. My wife might send me out to buy a half a dozen bagels. Sometimes I would buy a dozen, and eat six in the car on the way home. If I went out to dinner, I would order my meal and then wipe out an entire basket of bread prior to the arrival of the food. But sometimes even that wasn't enough—I would "reload"—I would ask the busboy to bring a second basket of bread, and I would put that second basket away as well!

No matter how much I ate during the meal—soup, salad, main course, vegetables, potatoes, you name it—there was always room for dessert, and maybe some of my wife's as well! And then when I got home, I'd still feel the urge to rummage around the kitchen. My urges would take me directly to the ice cream. I would hear that little voice inside that said, "Go ahead, Harry, you can have just a little."

I would heed that voice, telling myself that I was in control—that I could have a little bit of ice cream with no bad consequences. Of course, if you are a food addict and a binger like I am, you know where this is headed. A little bit of ice cream would lead to a little bit more, and then a little bit more, and before I knew it, I would have devoured an entire quart.

And then the next morning, I would get up, put on my suit and tie and my white doctor's lab coat, and return to my office at UCLA Medical Center, where I would warn my patients who were suffering from diabetes, high blood pressure, and high cholesterol of the dangers of overeating.

Clearly, something had to change.

The first thing that changed was that I started to learn about why people gain weight.

Your Body: Perfect for the Stone Age

The basic fact about weight gain is that we as a society eat too much. We no longer have to grow our food—we don't even have to cook it most of the time! We just go to the supermarket, put it in our cart, and often start eating it on the way home. This era of instant food gratification is something relatively new in human history. For thousands of years, our ancestors had to grow—or kill—what they ate. Their bodies were prepared to withstand long stretches when food would not be available in abundance. As a result, we as a species developed the ability to slow down our metabolism accordingly, similar to the way bears hibernate in the winter. Our bodies would be slow to metabolize the food that we ate, knowing that it might be a while before our next meal.

Today, though, there is an overabundance of food for those of us who live in the United States and other countries of the West. Food is always right around the corner. As a result, we tend to eat either a little bit more, or often far more, than we really need in order to run our bodies efficiently. The types of food that we eat, ironically enough, trigger the body's ancient starvation mentality. **The number one culprit in this area is starch—breads, pasta, pizza, cereal, rice, potatoes and the like.** The body figures that since it's being fed starch, there may not be any more food coming for a long time. So the more of the starch we eat, the more slowly the body metabolizes food, and the more weight we gain.

This occurs because starches are cheap and readily available foods that can be stored without refrigeration. Over the course of evolution, the body saw these as "storage" foods. For thousands of years before the invention of refrigeration, people couldn't store steak, chicken, or fish, or fruits, or vegetables. On the other hand, they *could* store flour for as long as a year without refrigeration, which meant that they could make bread and pasta whenever they wished. Rice and potatoes, also starch, were easy to store and did not need to be refrigerated.

As a result, when our ancestors ate starch, they sent a message to their bodies that nutritious, protein-rich foods like meat and fish, and simple carbohydrate foods like vegetables and fruits, simply would not be available. So their bodies acted wisely and slowed the metabolic rate, so as to preserve the calories—and energy—from those starch-based foods for as long as possible. The human body thus views the eating of anything made from starch—again, breads, pasta, pizza, cereal, rice, potatoes and the like—as a signal that hard times are coming, that no meat, vegetables, or fruit are likely to be available, and the body better "hang on" to the calories lest it starve.

Your body thinks it's doing you a colossal favor and actually protecting you from starvation. *You* know that there's plenty of meat, fruit, and vegetables in the fridge. But your body doesn't! And that's why starch is the easiest way to gain weight. Simply put, *starch is the signal to your body that you want to keep your weight where it is.* The body is programmed to try to keep its weight the same at all times—yo-yoing isn't healthy, and your body knows it. You can think of starch as the key device that affects your body's thermostat for burning food. If you eat starch, you are signaling your body that you do not want to lose weight.

If you *avoid* starch, then you are giving your body a very different signal indeed—that you *do* want to lose weight. Eliminate starch from your diet, which is the cornerstone of the *18% Solution*, and the unwanted excess weight will simply slide off.

If like many dieters you check the scale daily, you'll find nothing more discouraging than seeing your weight remain the same, or even rise, despite, all your hard work dieting. You can't afford to eat starch (or salt, for that matter) if you want to lose weight.

Let's talk about starch for a moment. The media, and most diet plans, claim that carbs are the problem when it comes to weight gain. Many diets urge dieters to ward off carbs completely, at least initially. We are bombarded in our popular culture today with messages that tell us that carbs are no good. Wherever we turn, we see "low carb" emblazoned on packages of food. We hear about all kinds of diets, diet aids, diet supplements, and the like, that all tout the benefits of a low carb or no carb lifestyle. And yet, even on an intuitive level, it doesn't make sense to most people who think about it that carbs could possibly be all bad.

Some carbs, like fruit and vegetables, are fine. But the carbs found in starchy foods, like breads, pasta, pizza, cereal, rice, potatoes and the like, only cause trouble if you're trying to lose weight.

Many dieters like to joke about being choc-aholics, people who never met a piece of chocolate they didn't like. It may come as a surprise that the number one food desired by people who tend to overeat or become obese isn't chocolate.

It's bread.

Breads, pasta, pizza, cereal, rice, potatoes and the like—those are the real problem. It's virtually impossible to lose weight, and virtually guaranteed to gain if a person continues to eat bread in any quantity. Even one piece of bread has the power to "lock up" weight loss for an entire week. So the heart of the *18% Solution* is to recognize that carbs in general are not the culprit—just starch. Starch triggers weight gain, pure and simple. Avoiding starch of any kind is the most important single change that an individual can make in order to cause a reduction in his or her weight.

How big a difference does starch make? Simply put, when you eat starch, you are slowing your metabolism down by one third. Your body will actually process food at a one third slower rate if it detects starch.

Let's take the example of Steve, who weighs around 175 pounds and consumes 1600 calories a day. If some of those calories come from starch, his metabolism will burn 1,600 calories a day. No weight gain, no weight loss. But if Steve eats those same 1,600 calories a day *avoiding* starch, his body will burn *2400* calories. In other words, avoiding starch gives your body the equivalent of a 33% head start in weight loss.

If Steve makes just one change to his diet—eliminating starch—and he still eats the exact same amount of food (replacing the starch with protein, vegetables, fruit, or anything else permitted on the diet), *he will lose approximately a pound and a half a week.*

Why is eliminating starch so incredibly important?

Let's do some caloric math together. Consider eating three oranges (60 calories per orange, or a total of 180 calories) versus one slice of pizza (170 calories for a slice of a nationally famous pizza home delivery chain's basic pizza.).

First of all, nobody eats just one slice of pizza! If you're having one slice, and if you're anything like me, chances are you're going to have two or three. So we're really talking about 340 calories, or even 510 calories, with three slices of pizza.

Three slices of pizza is pretty filling for most people, and that represents 510 calories, and yet we still might wash that pizza down with high-calorie soda or beer.

Three oranges are *extremely* filling for most people, and we've only consumed 180 calories.

510 vs. 180.

In addition, by avoiding starch, we burn one third more calories by keeping our metabolism up. Remember that eating starch reduces your metabolism by a third. Best of all, by avoiding starch, you're giving the body the signal that you really do want to drop the pounds.

Starch is the culprit. If you get rid of starch, the weight will slide away.

The Bran Muffin: The Stealth Bomber of Weight Gain

Why do so many people who exercise regularly and otherwise take great care of themselves find themselves gaining ten pounds a year?

Ironically enough, it all comes down to a single bran muffin.

What could be healthier than a bran muffin? Bran is healthy—we all know that because we heard it on TV. A bran muffin is a healthy, even virtuous choice when we are confronted with banana-nut muffins, chocolate cake, croissants, or the myriad of other baked goods that we find just about anywhere we go—from the coffee house on the corner to the gourmet restaurant downtown. There's only one problem with bran muffins—*they contain over 750 calories.*

I know that bran muffins are listed on various websites as containing only 375 calories … but that's 375 calories *per serving*, and the typical bran muffin actually contains two "servings"—not just one. So when you're ordering a bran muffin, you're saying hello to 750 fairly empty calories.

Let's do the math together. If you eat just one bran muffin a week—not daily but just *once a week*—you are adding 750 calories to your body every single week, calories it probably doesn't need. Over the course of a month, four bran muffins—just one a week, mind you—equals 3,000 calories per month. To gain a pound, you need to eat 3500 calories over and above your personal nutritional requirements. Just four bran muffins a month, at 750 calories per muffin, equals 3000 calories per month—or almost an entire pound of added body weight per month. And that's roughly ten pounds per year.

And that's just *one* bran muffin a week! Eat two or three a week, and it's good-bye, slim and attractive and hello, love handles, pot belly, and before too many years pass, obesity and all the health risks that come with carrying too much weight.

Of course, the great irony is that when people choose bran muffins over seemingly less healthy options, they think they are doing their bodies a great service. Five years and fifty pounds later, they might wonder exactly where all that excess weight came from, and that seemingly innocent bran muffin must take the blame.

By the way, a mile on a treadmill, as commendable as that may be, doesn't entitle a person to a big starch-filled meal, like a bagel and cream cheese or a bran muffin. Let's do the math. A typical 175-pound man burns up about 125 to 130 calories per mile on a treadmill. A woman who weighs 130 pounds burns less than 100 calories covering the same distance. Since muffins contain 750 calories, you'd have to walk or run more than six miles to burn off a single bran muffin!

Is eating a bran muffin worth running a 10K? I don't think so!

So there are two different ways to gain a great deal of weight. One way is to binge regularly, and overeat drastically. The way of the binger is a shortcut to rapid weight gain. But the epidemic of obesity in our society encompasses far more individuals than those who are addicted to overeating and bingeing. There is a second way people gain weight. People who generally take care of themselves, exercise, and eat fairly well are just as prone to becoming overweight or even grossly overweight—it just takes them a little bit longer, but the sad fact is that they get there nonetheless.

In many ways, I was both of these individuals. I was the binger who, once in a while, would put away those half dozen bagels on the way home from the bagel shop, the secret eater who would sneak into the kitchen and consume the carton of ice cream without ever saying a word to my wife. And at the same time, I was the virtuous eater (when other people were looking!) who would choose the bran muffin over the seemingly less healthy options when the choice arose.

So you could say that I gained weight both quickly *and* slowly! However I got there, the fact is that I did weigh 235 pounds, and I wasn't too proud of it, especially considering the fact that part of my work as a physician was to counsel individuals against weight gain.

Like most overweight people, I tried many diets. Like virtually all dieters, I had the same results—some degree of weight loss, followed by a pent-up craving for "forbidden" foods; which triggered relapse into overeating and bingeing, followed by weight gain that took me up past the original figure at which I had started the diet. Gaining and losing weight in itself is unhealthy. I found myself on the same diet/weight gain roller coaster that so many of my patients found themselves on—and could not get off.

There had to be a better way.

As a result, I looked more deeply into the question of why people gain weight, and I came up with a diet for myself. It is a well know fact that insulin resistance and obesity are linked. Obese people have insulin resistance. My theory is that starches trigger the insulin resistance response in obese people. Therefore I postulated that eliminating starches would result in weight loss. I had an abstract at the 2000 American Diabetes Association meeting which demonstrated the weight loss and lipid reduction on this diet. From that basic premise, I went on to develop and refine, partly by experimentation, and partly by observation the steps and stages of the 18% Solution diet.

On this diet that I designed for myself, I dropped sixty pounds in seven months, going from 235 pounds down to my current weight of around 175, plus or minus ten pounds (nobody stays at exactly the same weight all the time).

I have kept those sixty pounds off since 1998. The first person to notice my weight loss—aside from my wife, of course—was my next-door neighbor, who wanted to know how I did it. So I explained the basics of my diet to my neighbor. He went on the diet and dropped fifty pounds. My patients also noticed that they were seeing a slimmer and trimmer Harry Weisman, M.D., and they wanted to know what I was doing to get the weight off and keep it off. So I began to share some of the ideas of the diet with my patients. Gradually, more and more friends, family, and even other doctors started to ask me about the weight loss plan that I was using, so I shared the information with them.

Since 1998, I have shared my diet with hundreds of my patients, who range in age from adolescents to eighty-year-olds. Many of my diabetic patients who follow the diet have been able to go off insulin. Many of my cardiomyopathy patients have postponed the need for heart transplants. The diet works across the board, for people of every age, ethnic or racial background, and every socioeconomic level. If it worked for all of these people, it will surely work for you.

One trait that many overweight and truly obese people share is the fact that *they simply have no ideat what healthy eating looks like.* I think of one particular patient who came to me when he weighed 325 pounds. After five months on the diet, he had dropped sixty pounds, so he now weighed around 265 pounds—but he had begun to stop losing weight. I asked him if he was still following the diet, and he assured me that he was. As you'll see, the diet permits one meal every day with an unlimited amount of protein, and the diet also permits unlimited fruits and vegetables (despite what you may have heard, carbs *are* very good for you—as long as they are the right carbs!)

So I asked this patient what he was eating, because I wanted to know why he had plateaued at 265 pounds. He explained that his unlimited protein meal consisted of four steaks or six chicken breasts! His idea of "unlimited fruits" meant twenty-five fruits, every single day!

No wonder he wasn't losing any more weight!

I had to share with him a concept of what "reasonable" eating might be. Naturally, I couldn't ask him to go from a four-steak or six chicken breasts-a-day habit down to a single steak or chicken breast! I shared with him the reasons for limiting himself to a maximum of three steaks at one sitting each day, and just a few grapefruit instead of twenty-five to thirty. As a result, his weight loss began in earnest once again, and he is down in the low 240s at this writing.

Whether you are seriously overweight, like this gentleman, or whether you simply want to lose those eight or ten or fifteen last stubborn pounds once and for all, I can help you. The diet that I have shared with my neighbors, friends, family, patients, and colleagues will allow you to lose approximately 1% of your body weight every single week—so that after eighteen weeks, you will have lost more than 18% of your current weight. It worked for me, it works for my patients at the UCLA Medical Center, and it will absolutely work for you.

One of the beautiful things about the *18% Solution* is that you don't have to keep track of how many calories you eat. I'm much more interested in making sure that you eat foods that are healthy, filling, and nutritious. If you do that, and if you avoid starch, and the high fat foods and methods of food preparation that we will discuss, you are bound to lose 1% of your body weight each week.

Another important aspect of the *18% Solution* is that it takes into account the fact that *bingers cannot stop bingeing*. It's true that a foodaholic or a food addict can go without bingeing for a period of weeks or even sometimes months. But the medical fact is that people who binge are psychologically *bound* to binge, and there is absolutely no diet on the planet, no food plan, no prepared food from any company, that can possibly keep a binger from the psychological need to binge.

As a binger myself, I completely understand that state of mind. I had to create a diet that would work for me so that I would no longer have to deal with the consequences of all those excess calories. So my diet is completely binge-friendly.

I will never ask you to stop bingeing, contrary to just about every other diet on the market! Instead, I *will* ask you to substitute different types of foods for your binges, so that you are not doing your body any harm when you act out on that irrepressible urge to overeat.

If you are a food addict, you can't fight the feeling—and the great news is that you no longer have to. You can binge to your heart's content—as long as you binge on healthy foods. What are healthy foods? It may come as a great surprise to you in today's world where carbs are the culprits in most popular diet plans. On the *18% Solution*, however, you'll discover that some carbs—fruits and vegetables—are perfectly healthy and life-enhancing. The problem carbs are the starches—breads, pasta, pizza, cereal, rice, potatoes and the like. Understanding the difference between healthy and unhealthy carbs—or carbs that promote weight loss and carbs that prevent it—is at the heart of the diet plan.

There are three keys to the *18% Solution*, in addition to avoiding starch. Use these three keys and you'll lose all the weight you want … happily, easily, safely. You'll find each of the three keys defined and explained in the next chapter.

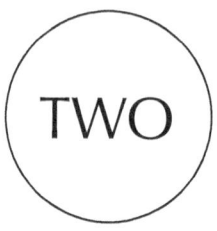

MEDICAL ISSUES AND
WEIGHT LOSS

The great news about the 18% Solution is that the program affords marvelous relief to those millions of individuals who suffer from diabetes, high cholesterol, hypertension, high blood pressure, heart disease, sleep apnea, polycystic ovaries, osteoarthritis, and reflux. When you adopt the 18% Solution, you don't just lose weight. You regain control over your health in extremely important ways, and this is great news both for you and for your family. Let's take a look at how the 18% Solution benefits sufferers from each of the diseases and conditions I mentioned above. Please note that each of the following are complex medical conditions requiring the care of a knowledgeable physician. I want to share with you the connection between being overweight and developing these illnesses, which are often reversible as you shed those excess pounds.

Diabetes

More than six percent of the U.S. population is diabetic, and of those individuals, ninety-five percent are Type II diabetics. These Type II diabetics are usually overweight and may or may not be taking insulin. The great news is that this type of diabetic responds dramatically to the 18% Solution. Diabetics are often weaned off insulin in a very short period of time. Those who are taking medication for poor glucose control can get their glucose under excellent control … and reduce the number of pills they must take. Several major studies have demonstrated conclusively that when diabetics attain good control of their glucose, it minimizes their complications of blindness and kidney disease.

High Cholesterol

High cholesterol is rampant in the United States. Several major studies have shown that those individuals who have previously suffered heart disease reduce their risk of a repeat bout of heart disease if they reduce their cholesterol. For those who are fortunate enough not to have suffered heart disease in the past, the 18% Solution will lower the risk of their ever experiencing heart disease in their lives. Within just one month, the 18% Solution typically lowers the cholesterol level in most people with significantly elevated cholesterol ... by at least twenty-five percent, and usually more, taking most of them to the normal range.

Hypertension

Hypertension is another epidemic in the United States. It is a major cause of heart disease, kidney disease, and strokes. All of these can be minimized by lowering blood pressure. The 18% Solution rapidly lowers blood pressure in a matter of weeks for most people who stick to the diet. My patients are typically able to reduce or even go off their hypertension medications altogether and improve their overall health.

Congestive Heart Failure—Cardiomyopathy

Insulin resistance, which is associated with obesity, contributes to cardiomyopathy and congestive heart failure. If you lose weight and embark on an exercise program, your heart health improves. The underlying heart disease does not go away, yet even those with heart disease attain a substantial improvement in the quality of their lives. Many of my patients who have been very overweight and have congestive heart failure or cardiomyopathy were unable to walk more than a block. With weight loss and exercise training, they now can walk more than a mile.

Sleep Apnea

Sleep apnea is a condition in which the individual experiences decreased respiration at night. This causes sleepiness during the day and also has a long-term deleterious effect on the heart. Individuals with sleep apnea often snore, disturbing their spouses. Many of those with sleep apnea can reverse its effects by losing weight. Daytime sleepiness and snoring are eliminated with weight loss. Sleep apnea sufferers often need a C-PAP machine to aid their nighttime breathing; weight loss can do away with the need for this device.

Osteoarthritis

The number one treatment for osteoarthritis is weight loss. Osteoarthritis is a disease in which the cartilage of joints, such as the hip and the knee, are eaten away. This leads to severe pain and the inability to walk or participate in sports. Those with osteoarthritis eventually need joint replacements. Studies have shown that weight loss reduces the symptoms of osteoarthritis, prevents further deterioration of the joints, and allows for greater participation in the activities of daily living.

Fatty Liver

A major cause of liver disease is a fatty liver. This can be caused by poor diabetic control, abnormally high lipids in the blood, or by obesity. All of these can be improved by weight loss. The 18% Solution at a minimum will lessen any liver abnormalities and often totally normalizes them.

Polycystic Ovary Disease

This disease is associated with abnormal menstrual periods, infertility, and abnormal hair growth. It is caused by insulin resistance. Weight loss reverses this syndrome.

Acid Reflux (GERD or Gastroesophageal Reflux Disease)

Millions of Americans suffer from acid reflux and know it by its more popular name, heartburn. Thus, millions of Americans take antacids and H2 blockers such as Tagamet and other drugs for this disease. When a patient modifies diet and loses weight, many of the symptoms of this very disabling disease can be alleviated.

◆   ◆   ◆

In short, the 18% Solution does a lot more than help you lose weight and keep the weight off. It alleviates a host of extremely serious medical conditions, granting you not just a healthy new body, but a healthy new life.

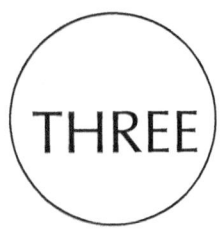

THREE

THE 3 KEYS TO THE 18% SOLUTION

In this chapter, I'd like to introduce you to the three keys to the *18% Solution*: drink plenty of water; eat plenty of fruit; and get out and walk. Let's take a look at why each of these keys is so important.

Key 1: Drink Plenty of Water!

Drink a *lot* of water! Specifically, I want you to drink at least two quarts or approximately two liters, the equivalent of eight eight-ounce glasses of water *every single day*.

You can drink bottled or tap water, as you choose—just don't drink carbonated water. Most Americans are simply dehydrated. We don't get enough water, which is actually the single most perfect thing we can consume to re-energize ourselves and reinvigorate our bodies. A side benefit: when you drink a lot of water, you're not as hungry for food, as water is an excellent curb for our appetites.

When we diet, our bodies excrete a lot of liquid. If this liquid is not replaced, we will experience dizziness, weakness, irritability, and fatigue. Drinking lots of liquids fills us up and thereby prevents malaise. Adequate liquid consumption also tends to prevent constipation.

We often misread a signal from our body indicating a desire for water, and we think that actually we need to eat something. For that reason, we eat, in order to counteract a feeling of sluggishness. Ironically, eating makes us feel more sluggish … which makes us feel like eating more … which makes us even more sluggish

… and so on, until our energy level is depleted. Drinking water keeps us energized and reduces that urge to eat.

Another reason why water is so important: for our ancestors, water was an essential part of their diet, but it was awfully hard to find. And yet the human body *needs* salt and water in balance, in order to keep literally millions of functions working. If our forebears didn't get enough water, they would eat salt in order to retain water. This was another protective device that the human body employed in order to keep from shutting down.

Today, we retain water just as easily as our ancestors did. Eating salt causes water retention. The only difference is that we aren't stranded in the desert—we're living in modern society. During times of starvation as well, the body gets dehydrated. It adjusts by retaining water and salt. The body makes the salt more potent in retaining water. What does this mean for your body?

Your body is actually trying to help you, by making the water last as long as it can. So when we don't drink enough water, our consumption of salt causes an enhanced amount of water retention! And this leads to serious weight gain.

Our ancestors didn't drink enough water because they often didn't have access to it. We "moderns" aren't getting enough water, because we often don't realize the importance of drinking enough of it. Whatever the reason for not drinking enough water, the result is always the same: low circulatory volume, causing increased salt effect and water retention. There is a proven relationship between salt intake water retention, and weight gain. The bottom line: drink more water, retain less salt, lose more weight.

No Drinking While Eating!

Don't drink any water half an hour before, with, or after any meal. Diluting food in the stomach delays the transit time of the food. It allows more time for the absorption of calories. Also, when we drink while we eat, we may become distracted from just how much food we are consuming—and we are likely to eat more food than necessary in order to satiate ourselves. So don't drink before, during or after meals—one half hour in either direction. When you have to wait half an hour, you're far more likely to be conscious of when you will eat and how much food you will eat. It's harder to graze, nibble, or snack if you're being careful to drink plenty of water and to eat only when there is a thirty-minute gap from the time you last had water to drink.

What to Drink, What Not to Drink

On the *18% Solution*, I want you to avoid beverages that do not support weight loss. First, I don't want you to have any fruit or vegetable juice, fresh, canned, or frozen. The juicing process allows the water, color, and sugar to come out of the fruit into the juice. This makes the sugar in the juice too easily absorbable for the body to handle the sugar load efficiently. This sets up unhealthy insulin levels, which produce a vicious cycle of the body going into starvation mode. On top of that, juices are not very filling. There is just simply too much sugar and salt in these juices for your well-being. They are not permitted, because they are not a wise nutritional choice.

You may drink diet soda on the *18% Solution*—but I don't encourage it. There's no sugar in diet soda, but you do have all kinds of chemicals and often salt. That's why I don't encourage diet soda. On the *18% Solution*, you can have one can of diet soda daily—maximum.

You may drink unsweetened tea, either cold or hot. I would prefer that you drink decaffeinated or herbal tea. That's because caffeine dehydrates the body.

You may drink coffee, either hot or iced. Decaffeinated or herbal coffee substitutes are preferred, for the same reason. With your coffee, you cannot use any of the following: sugar, whiteners, creamers, powders, soy milk, half and half or mocha mix. That's because they either contain a high concentration of sugar or unhealthy fats.

You may use Sweet 'n Low, Equal or Splenda, and you may add up to one half ounce of non-fat milk per cup of coffee.

Here comes the bad news. If you are a lover of beer, wine, cosmopolitans, martinis, or any other form of alcoholic beverage—in the early stages, the *18% Solution* permits no wine, no beer, and no liquor of any kind.

Drinking alcohol is absolutely incompatible with the initial phase of any weight loss reduction plan. (There is light at the end of the tunnel—don't empty out your wine cellar! Just avoid it until you reach the maintenance phase!)

You can eat all the vegetables you want on the *18% Solution*, but don't cook the vegetables—or fruits, for that matter. That's because cooking alters the chemical makeup of the cell walls of fruits and vegetables, allowing more sugar to be easily absorbed. The energy required by the body to digest the hard food or vegetable is no longer expended. To see this for yourself, think about how long it takes to eat a crunchy raw carrot and how hard it is to digest that, compared with eating a soft cooked carrot that even a baby can easily digest. Cooked vegetables and fruits are not permitted, because eating them won't help you lose weight.

All You Can Eat!

There was a wonderful syndicated columnist named Mike Royko who once published in one of his newspaper columns the "Mike Royko Diet," which was his satirical response to the many diet crazes that were sweeping the nation. On the Mike Royko Diet, whatever you liked, you couldn't eat at all. But whatever you hated, you could eat to your heart's content!

Royko's satire points up a key fact about dieting—the sense of deprivation invariably leads to a massive need for bingeing. In order to help you feel completely satiated, and to avoid that feeling of deprivation, *you can eat all you want of the permitted foods on the 18% Solution.* I want this eating plan to be a luxurious experience for you! Enjoying a filet mignon with endives, a gourmet salad and having mango, star fruit, or raspberries for dessert—that doesn't sound like deprivation to me!

I hope you don't interpret this to mean that you can eat 25 grapefruits a day, the way the patient I mentioned earlier did. But everything has to be put into perspective. Even twenty-five grapefruits is a big step up from 25 donuts, or 25 bagels, or 25 pastries.

Key 2: Eat Plenty of Fruit

On the *18% Solution*, you can have all the fruit you want.

It is difficult to feel psychologically deprived when you're permitted to eat unlimited amounts of steak (see chapter 6) and all the exotic and regular fruits you like. If you're going to binge (and if you are a binge-prone individual, like me, there is no avoiding bingeing), it's so much better for you to binge on fruit than on ice cream, candy, or, worst of all, bread or any other starch.

On this diet plan, the energy you need to get through your day comes from fruit. When you eat fruit, the energy you gain lasts about three hours. If you don't eat fruit every three hours, irritability, fatigue, listlessness and hunger set in. Eating fruit less than six times per day is not a good idea for anyone on the *18% Solution*.

However, dried fruit, like raisins, dates, figs, apricots, bananas, are not permitted on the diet. Drying fruits alters their chemical makeup, so that more sugar is absorbed when they are eaten. In addition, sugar is absorbed more quickly, because the sugar is now more concentrated. It is easier to eat twenty dried apricots than to eat twenty fresh apricots—and much less filling. Dried fruits are not permitted, for these reasons.

Fruit is extremely attractive to the eye and to the taste buds. The more you study the nutritional value of fruit, the more you see that fruit is one of nature's most perfect foods. And yet, most low carb or no carb diets permit little to no fruit. On the *18% Solution*, you'll be able to enjoy all the fruits and vegetables you like.

If you binge, then binge on fruit and/or vegetables most of the time. Binge occasionally on hard-boiled eggs. But don't binge on high calorie foods like ice cream, chocolate, candy, or starches, or any of the other foods to which bingers naturally gravitate.

Key 3: Get Out and Walk!

On the *18% Solution*, it is absolutely necessary to exercise DAILY. Most of us are absolute couch potatoes—the average exercise performed by the average American consists of reaching for the remote control and going channel surfing. Our thumbs are probably the healthiest parts of our bodies!

On the *18% Solution*, I don't advocate any sort of strenuous exercise, for a variety of reasons. First, many of the people who go on this diet are grossly overweight—so it would not be a healthy recommendation for people in that category to suddenly start jogging. Second, walking is just about the most healthful exercise that anyone can do. You don't need to belong to a fancy gym, you don't need equipment, you don't need a partner, and you don't need a trainer. You do need a good pair of walking or running shoes, though.

Anybody can find a place to walk. Recently on the news, one of the Vietnam veterans who had been held hostage in the "Hanoi Hilton" told reporters that he was able to walk twelve miles a day—in a six foot by eight foot cell. If he can cover that sort of distance under those conditions, certainly you can find a time and place for walking, too!

I'm not asking you to walk anything near twelve miles a day. This chart explains exactly how much I want you to walk on each day of the diet. You'll be starting at one mile per day and increasing your walk by a quarter of a mile each week until you reach three miles a day.

THE *18% SOLUTION* EXERCISE PLAN

WEEK	DISTANCE
First Week	Walk 1 mile per day
Second Week	Walk 1 ¼ miles per day.
Third Week	Walk 1 ½ miles per day.
Fourth Week	Walk 1 ¾ miles per day.
Fifth Week	Walk 2 miles per day.
Sixth Week	Walk 2 ¼ miles per day.
Seventh Week	Walk 2 ½ miles per day.
Eighth Week	Walk 2 ¾ miles per day.
Ninth Week	Walk 3 miles per day. Thereafter, walk at least 3 miles per day.

You can walk around your neighborhood, around your office building if you work in an office, at the beach, at a park, wherever you like. If the weather is not conducive to walking outside, you can always walk in a mall or on a treadmill. The main thing is to get your walking in, no matter what. We've got to get our bodies moving in order to get rid of that excess weight. Walking burns calories and, just as important, it also increases our metabolism.

Those are the three keys to the diet—drink plenty of water, eat plenty of fruit, and get out and walk. In the next chapter, I'll show you exactly how to implement the *18% Solution* in your own life, so you can begin to enjoy the benefits of permanent weight loss. So let's get started!

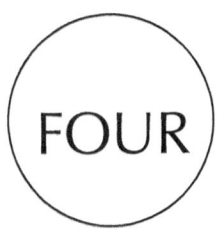

FOUR

MAKING THE PROGRAM
WORK FOR YOU

Every body is different. So there is no "one size fits all" way to use the 18% Solution. The plan does have three phases, and each phase has a series of different stages. You'll go through each of the stages of each phase in your own way and pace, so that the program is most comfortable for you. The speed at which you will progress from one stage to another, and from one phase to another of the plan, depends on a variety of factors—how much weight you wish to lose, the degree to which you follow the guidelines, your own goals, and the uniqueness of your own body.

Let's first discuss the three phases of the plan. I call phase one "Cleansing and Relearning," because in this phase, you will be removing all the toxins from your system and replacing them with healthier foods and beverages, and you will essentially be relearning how to eat! Eating seems like the most natural thing in the world—after all, we just reach for some food and we put it in our mouths. Yet learning to eat in a healthy manner is quite different. Most of us did not learn how to "eat healthy" while we were children. This is not about blaming our parents—the information that I'm sharing with you today simply was not known back when you and I were growing up. Our parents were always doing the best they could, based on the information they had available at the time. You could say the same thing about us, as well! We were always doing the best we could, based on the information we had. Well, today I'm here to provide you with better information, so that you can eat better, live healthier, happier, and longer. And the first step in this process is to cleanse your system and "relearn" the optimal way of providing yourself the nutrition—and the enjoyment!—that good food provides.

The second phase is all about losing weight. Once we've gotten our systems clean and healthy, it's now time to begin the weight loss phase of the program in a carefully managed way. As I've said elsewhere, this is not a Hollywood diet, or a fad diet, or a "lose weight to look good in the wedding pictures" kind of diet. This is really about reshaping your relationship with food, so that you are nourishing yourself and replenishing your body with all the nutrients and power it needs to maximize your energy and help you enjoy your day to the fullest. I've been working with patients at UCLA for close to thirty years as an endocrinologist, so the information and plans I will share with you for weight loss are safe, thoroughly tested, and, best of all, effective. They really work.

After you've lost the weight you intend to lose—in a measured and healthy manner—we move to the third phase of the program, the Maintenance Phase. So many of us have been on "yo-yo diets"—where our weight goes down … and then back up … and then down again … and then up again … and unfortunately, we seem to add a few pounds every time we go up. Well, that's why I've included this maintenance phase, which has worked wonderfully for my patients—and for myself. So many of us tend to "reward ourselves" when we lose weight … by reverting to our prior, unhealthy eating habits, and putting the weight back on. Or perhaps we self-sabotage—for whatever reason, we can't stand the idea that we have actually become thinner and more attractive, and so we find ourselves eating not to nourish ourselves, but to put ourselves back in the unhappy position of being overweight … simply because it's familiar. Adhering to the maintenance phase of the 18% Solution will put all that in the past for you. I will share with you a method for maintaining your weight loss not just for a few weeks or months but for the rest of your life, and after all, isn't that our real goal? I never want you to have to lose that weight again!

Healthy adults who want to lose weight and increase their health and well-being can follow this diet on their own without medical supervision. This diet is not appropriate for pregnant women, women who are nursing, type I diabetics, and individuals with chronic renal disease. People with other illnesses must check with their physician first and be under his/her supervision.

Will the 18% Solution work for me?

The 18% Solution is expressly indicated for individuals with type II diabetes, congestive heart failure, and hypertension, as long as they go onto the plan with close physician supervision. I recommend at least weekly visits in your initial period on the 18% Solution. Close physician contact is crucial because you will need frequent blood tests in the first few weeks, to adjust the medications downward: blood pressure medications, heart medications, water pills, blood thinners (Coumadin), oral diabetic medications, and insulin. If the only benefit of the 18% Solution was that you got to reduce or even eliminate these medications, that might be enough for a lot of people!

In order to get started, I suggest that you familiarize yourself with the general guidelines of the 18% Solution, which apply to all phases of the plan. These include the suggestions I will offer throughout the book with regard to exercise, supplements, condiments, and beverages, and they constitute the basic requirements of a healthy lifestyle. You definitely want to adhere to these suggestions on a daily basis for the rest of your life.

I'll offer you an entire chapter on exercise. To summarize the suggestions you will find there, I want you to walk at any speed that is comfortable for you, preferably slowly at first, on a street, track, treadmill, or in a shopping mall. I'll be asking you to increase by a quarter of a mile the amount you walk each week until you reach at least three miles per day. It is vital to walk every day. This walking is in addition to any other exercise that you do.

Supplements—I suggest that you take a multivitamin every day. Everyone should! It's best, also, to be taking 500 milligrams of calcium three times a day with meals. You can choose any source of calcium that you like—chewable Tums, Os-Cal, calcium carbonate, or calcium citrate. In addition, women who menstruate should take an iron pill daily. If you are over forty-five, it's best to take at least one baby aspirin every day to prevent stroke and heart disease, if you do not have a contraindication to aspirin.

Condiments—You may use any condiment or herb which is fresh and not packaged while you are on the 18% Solution. As for processed condiments, I want you to avoid all of the following, because they promote weight gain, water retention, or otherwise interfere with weight loss. They include salt, sugar, honey, mayonnaise, ketchup, any kind of oil (including olive oil), soy sauce, barbecue sauce, or salsa. You also need to avoid canned foods, frozen foods, and bottled foods, because they contain high quantities of salt, which promotes water retention.

Beverages—On the 18% Solution, it is necessary to drink two liters, approximately two quarts, of water every single day. This works out to about eight 8-ounce glasses of water. Avoid caffeine and carbonated beverages—caffeine dehydrates you, and most of us tend to think we're hungry when we're actually just thirsty! So while there may not be any calories in coffee, it may surprise you to learn that coffee makes you hungry, because caffeine is an appetite stimulant. You want to avoid carbonated beverages for two reasons: the carbonic acid, which produces the bubbles, stimulates your appetite, and these beverages also usually contain salt. If you choose to drink decaffeinated coffee, don't use half and half, soy milk, powders, or other creamers. Instead, you may only put in Sweet 'n' Low, Equal, or Splenda, and a little non-fat milk.

Guidelines for using the three phases and the stages of the 18% Solution

Let's take a deeper look at each of the phases and the stages of the 18% Solution. As we discussed, phase one consists of cleansing and relearning how to eat. I will share with you two strongly recommended stages for this phase and two optional stages. Definitely do the two recommended stages, Stage A and Stage B. Start with Stage A. Most people stay on it for at least four weeks. If you lose at least seven percent of your initial weight in four weeks, then you have mastered Stage A, and you are ready to move on. Some people only need a week or so on Stage A if the weight they need to lose represents less than ten percent of their overall body weight. Those who need to lose more weight will spend more time—usually a month—on this Stage.

Next comes Stage B, also for four weeks for most people. If you lose at least four percent of your weight in those four weeks, you've mastered Stage B and it's time to move on. Less weight to lose means less time on this stage as well.

I'd like to share with you some variations that some of my patients have opted for during phase one. These work just as well as the standard approach. In one variation, people can start with Stage AA for the first month, and then move to Stage A for the second month, and Stage B for the third month. Stage AA is more restrictive than Stage A. Some people prefer fewer choices to get started, and I certainly can understand why—sometimes it's easier to get started when there are fewer options. Whether you start with Stage A, or with the more restrictive Stage AA, or Stage B, is entirely a matter of your own personality and your personal style. Your weight loss results will be the same.

Another option to consider is Stage X. Whenever you are on this plan, regardless of what phase or stage you were on, you may always substitute up to five or six days per month of Stage X. The only time to declare a "Stage X day" is in the morning, when the day begins, and you must stick to it for at least one full day. It is not permissible on the 18% Solution to take a Stage X day more than seven times in four weeks.

Let's say you've tried Stage A *and* Stage B, and you find that you really cannot do either comfortably. If you've given them an honest try, then go directly to phase two, the weight loss phase. Everyone is unique, so don't hesitate to individualize the program to suit your particular needs. The main thing is never to give up!

Phase Two

Phase two of the 18% Solution is the Controlled, Healthy Weight-Loss Phase. I'll provide you with two recommended stages and one optional stage for this phase. Everyone should do the two recommended stages, Stage C and Stage D. There are special circumstances under which you can do the optional stage, Stage X.

Start with Stage C, and stick to it for four weeks. If you've lost at least four percent of your initial weight in those four weeks, you've mastered Stage C, and it's time to move on. Again, if you have less weight to lose, you'll spend less time here, as well.

After Stage C, it's time to advance to Stage D, and again, this stage usually lasts for four weeks. If you lose at least four percent of your weight in those four weeks, then you've mastered Stage D … and it's time once again to move on.

As in the first phase, Cleansing and Relearning to Eat, you can use Stage X anytime during this phase as well. The same rules apply—start in the morning, and stick to it for at least one full day, and limit your Stage X days to no more than seven days in the four-week period.

Phase Three

Phase three of the 18% Solution is the Maintenance Phase. Here you'll find eight recommended stages, starting with Stage E and going all the way through to Stage L. You've also got optional Stage X at your disposal throughout phase three. Please do the stages in order.

If you have not yet attained your goal weight by the time you've reached the maintenance phase, that's perfectly fine. Measure your progress this way: in every month when you have lost four percent of your weight, proceed to the next stage. If you have not lost four percent of your weight in one month, drop back a stage. It's not about winning or losing or completing the program in a new world record time! Again, it's about adjusting the 18% Solution so that it fits you, your body, your needs, and your goals.

Soon you will have attained your goal weight. Once at your goal weight, proceed to the next stage as long as you have lost more than one percent of your weight during the month. At any stage in the program, if you are losing less than one percent of your total body weight during a given month, you know that you have reached the maximum amount of food that your body can tolerate. If you eat more, you'll gain weight.

Keep in mind that Stage X is always an option for you as you go through phase three, the Maintenance Phase. And as before, only start a Stage X day in the morning, stick to it for at least one full day, and limit your Stage X days to no more than seven over the course of every four weeks.

Finally, let me share with you the concept of the "controlled cheat." You are entitled to a "controlled cheat" one day a month after the first month. You can eat anything you want from Stage L for one meal. This will give you a taste of freedom, and show you where you're headed. I always suggest to my patients that they use this "controlled cheat" for special occasions like birthdays and holidays, but only if they need to do so. It's not obligatory. This way, you'll see that there truly is light at the end of the diet tunnel!

Now you know the "rules of the game" for the 18% Solution ... so let's get started!

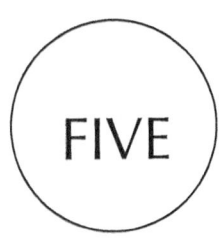

FIVE

THE POWER OF POSITIVE BINGEING

Let us define bingeing as eating when you are not truly hungry or eating more than you require in order to satiate hunger. You can binge on any kind of food, and on any amount of food, but most people binge on high fat foods, like ice cream, or starches like bread. If you eat soon after a good-sized meal, you are bingeing, since you cannot really be hungry in the normal sense of the term—your body doesn't require nourishment, and yet you feel the need to eat, and eat a lot.

People who binge—the foodaholics of the world—are usually prone to being overweight. Some binge daily and others binge occasionally. Lean people who are not foodaholics rarely binge.

There are many rationales and triggers for bingeing, *but none are related to hunger*. Bingeing is compulsive behavior reflecting a wide range of psychological needs. Each binger's profile is unique, as we are all unique individuals with unique histories and life situations. Yet, after treating many bingers, I have noticed some common patterns and motivations.

Anxiety is probably the number one trigger for bingeing. People often binge at social events such as high-pressure business meals, family functions, or cocktail parties, where they might be feeling some social stress or discomfort. We all experience stress and anxiety, but only food addicts—foodaholics—act out on stress and anxiety with bingeing.

Surprisingly, boredom often leads to bingeing. Boredom is often a state of high anxiety—because we don't know what to do with ourselves! In a restaurant, while waiting to order, or while waiting for the meal to be served, the binger often goes through one or more baskets of bread (I already admitted to this behavior in Chapter One!). Initially, the binger might have been truly hungry, but that would only explain the first slice of bread—not the four or six or ten that followed out of boredom.

Another example of eating while bored is while watching television or at the movies. Since adults typically watch television or go to the movies after dinner, it's unlikely that the snacks we consume are intended to satisfy hunger. The real reason we're eating when we're physically full: *eating relieves boredom.* The binger, anxious for the movie to start, gets a box of popcorn and most likely finishes it before the end of the "coming attractions." At home, the binger waits for the commercials to interrupt the TV program, goes to the kitchen, and gets more food which will be consumed in time for the next commercial/ food break.

Many of us binge when we are disappointed, as a way of soothing ourselves and attempting to fill a sense of emptiness. A student who does poorly on a test, an employee who does not get a promotion, an investor who loses on a transaction, or a suitor who is stood up may binge with the psychological rationale that says, "I deserve a treat in order to pick myself up."

Sometimes we binge as a way to retaliate against people whom we feel have hurt us. We eat, thinking to ourselves, "I'll show them." The implication is that those other people must really care about what we do to ourselves, and that the other person will feel guilty or remorseful because of the harm we cause ourselves. An exaggerated form of this behavior is the person who attempts suicide in order to punish someone else.

Despite the fact that we live in an affluent society, with an abundance of food everywhere, we are internally programmed to worry that if we do not stock up on food *right now*, we will starve. Before the binger boards a cross country flight, he or she will buy and bring on board a ton of food—in case there is a delay with the food service. Overeating at a smorgasbord preceding a full dinner is another example of this sense of "there won't be enough later."

In sum, we often eat out of habit and psychological need—and not because we are hungry. We may have completed a large breakfast or mid-morning snack at 11:00 a.m., but when everyone goes to lunch at noon, we will eat a full meal again.

Bingeing is often a partner with procrastination. Searching for, preparing, and eating food for which we are not really hungry is a very popular stalling device to keep people from focusing on unpleasant tasks such as preparing tax returns, getting important papers together, doing homework, and the like. People commonly binge when they have to meet a deadline. Most of us would rather nurture ourselves with food than confront an unpleasant or difficult task.

Anatomy of a Binge

There are many reasons why a person who binges feels bad. The binger feels that he does not have strong enough will power to resist temptation and stay in control—and therefore is not a person of strong character. A binger may feel he is always going to be a loser, and this is just another situation where he has lost. He may feel hopeless that he will always be fat, and feel helpless as well, because "nothing seems to work." A binger might also feel tired and sluggish because the foods on which he typically binges are foods with a high starch and high fat content—and these chemically cause fatigue.

Bingeing perpetuates bingeing in a vicious cycle leading to weight gain and low self-esteem. This cycle is perpetuated not only because of the increased calories consumed, but because the binge foods are typically high in starch and fat. These foods also cause a chemical reaction, which increases insulin and promotes *rapid* weight gain. Once a binger has gained so much weight so quickly, he rationalizes that he might as well keep on bingeing. What's the point of trying to diet and fail yet again? This individual has given up. Feeling like a failure keeps the binger depressed … and eating more.

Don't Fight the Feeling!

Fighting the urge to binge doesn't work. You can fight it for so long—but ultimately you will give in and binge. "I'll only binge this once" also does not work. Bingeing triggers a loss of self esteem and a sense of helplessness that there is no point in continuing to diet. It just doesn't work to binge "a little." Bingeing is like any other addiction—a chemical reinforcement exists, triggering the individual to continue the unhealthy behavior. It's time to stop applying value judgments to bingeing.

Bingeing may not be so bad.

The positives of bingeing actually make an impressive case! Bingeing helps keep the psyche of foodaholics in balance. It keeps them from feeling deprived because they associate nurturing with eating—a learned behavior from infant feeding. In addition, the instinct of the infant to suck, which once soothed us, remains as an oral fixation which is now expressed through eating. In short, bingeing may not be a behavior which needs to be stopped. In fact we would probably fail if we tried to stop it. Like many other behaviors, it simply needs to be channeled in a positive direction.

How do you channel that bingeing energy? First, you want to be aware of the times when bingeing is most likely. Let's review them:

1. When you are alone or watching TV.

2. While waiting for someone or waiting in a restaurant.

3. While waiting for news on an important decision.

4. Stressful situations, such as parties or business meetings.

5. After hearing disappointing news, in particular connected to a sense of personal failure or rejection.

6. When a deadline needs to be met, and there is much tension and a desire to procrastinate.

7. To "show someone"—by hurting yourself.

8. Late at night, or when overtired, and our normal defenses are down.

9. In an environment when others are bingeing—negative peer pressure.

10. On vacation or any other special occasion while feeling a sense of entitlement.

11. When you have started the day depressed and "give up" for that day, week, month, or year.

I want you to learn to recognize these "binger harbinger" signals. When one of those eleven situations occurs, and you find yourself heading to the refrigerator or pantry, thinking about food, or getting bored, a binge is coming on. What should you do about it?

Remember when you last binged, and it didn't matter what junk food was in the cupboard? It didn't even matter whether you liked it or not. You just ate it, in an out of control way. Instead, now channel that desire to binge toward healthy foods.

Binge to your heart's content on permitted foods—fruits and vegetables. The key to successful bingeing is to be *prepared* for positive bingeing. This means that you must maintain a constant supply of fruits and vegetables at home, at work, on trips, in your car, or wherever you go.

Most people find that the best food of all on which to binge is grapefruit! Others prefer oranges or melons, and those are fine as well. The sugars in fruit will fulfill your sense of craving. Almost any fruit will do.

If you binge on permitted foods such as fresh fruit or vegetables, you are staying on the *18% Solution*! You are not cheating! Even though you stay in control and do not go off the diet, you will have nurtured your psyche—because you binged, and you fulfilled your psychological need to chew. Bingeing on the permitted foods will even improve your mood. That's because in chemical terms, these foods trigger high energy—and not depression. So enjoy those fruits and vegetables to any degree you choose!

If you binge on prohibited foods, *stop right away.* Don't say "Once I have broken the diet, I am off it forever." The sooner you stop bingeing on the wrong foods and the sooner you get back on the *18% Solution*, the sooner you will begin to feel better about yourself—and the less weight you will have to lose.

A lot of people wonder whether there really is such a thing as food addiction, since all of us have to eat. The simple answer: yes.

Addictions come in many varieties. People who are addiction-free often have difficulty understanding how addicted people feel a loss of self control and free choice when confronted with the substance of their addiction. Obese people have a food addiction. More specifically, they suffer a food addiction to specific foods, which aggravates their problem and strengthens the addiction.

Addiction is a chemical need, triggered by certain receptors in the body which send out messages, dictating that the body obtain more of a specific substance. This addiction is genetic and is activated every time the body comes in contact with the triggering substance. Addiction is forever—people can arrest their addictions by avoiding the addictive substances or behaviors, but there is no such thing as turning an addict into a non-addict. As they say in Alcoholics Anonymous, you can't go back to being a cucumber once you've become a pickle!

Everyone recognizes addictions to cigarettes, alcohol, narcotics, and even caffeine. We understand that these are chemical addictions. When a person has any addiction to one or more of these substances, that person no longer has free choice over moderating or limiting consumption of the addicting substance. When an addict consumes the first drink of alcohol, he becomes unable to stop, no matter what the consequences to himself, his family, or others around him. He will continue to drink even if it costs him his job, his marriage, and his family. This is just as true for the drug addict, the nicotine addict … or the food addict.

Breaking the Cycle

Once an addict recognizes that he does not have free choice for his addiction, then the treatment strategy can be developed. The general protocol for the alcoholic, drug addict, nicotine addict or caffeine addict is to abstain totally in order to be successful. But food addicts cannot abstain totally from food—we have to continue to eat in order to survive. We therefore must be more precise in the case of the food addict and determine which foods are nutritious and safe in terms of not triggering the addiction cycle.

The *18% Solution* is based on the premise that the culprit for food addicts is starch. The more starch the food addict eats, the more he covets them and eats them in increasing quantities, and the more the vicious cycle spins. As the person becomes fatter, his metabolism slows down, and there is increasing deposition of fat on his body. He becomes hungrier—and eats even more. The fatter he gets, the higher his cholesterol goes. Eventually, he may develop other complications of obesity—specifically diabetes and high blood pressure.

It becomes obvious that the food addict must totally abstain from starch. Even a small amount of starch can activate the cycle—just as one taste of alcohol will trigger the alcoholic cycle. Think about it: What food addict can eat one single potato chip, or one french fry.

There is also a psychological component to addiction. Once in the cycle, the addict feels hopelessly caught in the web—and helpless to break free. He does not wish to risk the little self-esteem he has left in order to try and break that vicious cycle, lest he fail yet again. He becomes resigned to the addiction and its consequences. This is true for the alcoholic, and the narcotic addict—and it is equally true for the food addict. All of these addicts live in a state of resignation and hopelessness, which in turn engenders a state of depression.

If you consider yourself a food addict, I can help you break that cycle of low self esteem, helplessness and hopelessness. I can administer for you a powerful, effective, dramatic, and massive dose of positive reinforcement!

All you have to do is make a contract with me that you will commit to my program one hundred percent for one week. If you do, you will experience results that will trigger your own free will to desire to continue. In one week, you can break the vicious cycle and you can gain increased self esteem. In addition to having broken the chemical dependence on starch—and its deleterious effect on your health. Just as with the alcohol or narcotic addict, however, you have to comply one hundred percent in order to realize meaningful, lasting results.

There is no magic bullet to cure the alcoholic or the narcotic addict. Similarly, there is no magic bullet to cure the food addict. It takes motivation and hard work to be successful—and proper guidance, too. Most addicts hope and search for the miracle which will allow them to indulge in moderation—but it does not exist. The addict who successfully overcomes his addiction understands this, and realizes that abstinence is a way of life. The addict knows that it takes a commitment to live this way of life twenty-four hours a day, seven days a week, fifty-two weeks a year, with no exceptions. Despite attending a birthday party or wedding. Despite the wine being such a great vintage. Despite the social embarrassment or pressure to eat. The food addict requires the same commitment to successfully avoid starch twenty-four hours a day, seven days a week, fifty-two weeks a year just like the alcoholic or drug addict.

Similarly, the food addict who is committed to stopping must stop today—not next week. Addicts never taper off—they taper on! There are always a myriad of reasons why an addict should postpone starting the diet. These same reasons can be given tomorrow, and the next day as well. It's possible to rationalize why one need never start the diet. The best way—the only way—is to start right away.

The decision to start is an important first step, but it is just the beginning. As with any change, the beginning is hard, but eventually things get easier. As with the sober alcoholic, the food addict cannot become lax in his vigilance. Even if he is successful for months or years, he must always be aware of his food addiction. The routine of eating in a healthy manner and the positive reinforcement from all the benefits, including better health, better appearance, less medication should make it easier to continue. However, the food addict's best hope is to become a health addict—in a positive cycle of control, choice, high energy, and self esteem. Again, this M.D.'s best advice—start now! Eat to live, don't live to eat.

And that will result in your weight dropping. It's that simple.

On the *18% Solution*, you'll be able to enjoy an unlimited serving of protein every day (although I hope you won't use that as a license to eat four to six steaks and all those chicken breasts like the patient I mentioned earlier!). You'll be able to enjoy all the fruit and vegetables you wish. You'll be able to binge without feeling guilty—and without doing your health, or your waistline, any harm.

As a result, you will not feel that sense of deprivation that most diets create. When a dieter feels deprived, it's only a matter of time before some external event—bad news, good news, a raise, getting fired—sets off what you could call the "mother of all binges." That's why people gain back even more weight than they lost—they are reacting to the intense feelings of deprivation that lasted for the length of the diet. And then they feel even more despair, because all that hard work has now been for naught. On top of the despair, they feel the sense of failure and hopelessness—if this diet didn't work, then no diet ever will, and they will be doomed forever to be overweight, looking and feeling unattractive, and a prey to the wide range of health issues that being overweight entails.

That's why I say that this diet is safe, easy, and satisfying for the dieter—because there are no feelings of deprivation. You do get to eat as much as you want, pretty much as often as you want. I'm asking you to swear off breads, pasta, pizza, cereal, rice, potatoes and the like, and especially those seductive bran muffins! Giving up foods that do nothing for your health, well-being, or appearance is a small price to pay for looking and feeling great!

We will come back to this question of how weight loss really happens, and how the plan really works, but let's turn to some of the other concepts that underlie the *18% Solution* … in the next chapter.

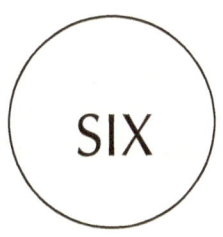

SIX

GETTING GOING WITH THE 18% SOLUTION

Check with your physician first.

Check with your physician before starting this eating and exercise plan, just as you should check with your physician before starting any eating or exercise plan. Explain to your physician that this is a low fat, no starch diet, and that you are permitted fruits, vegetables and protein. Tell your physician that the exercise I recommend is walking—in gradually increasing amounts.

Depending on your age and past medical history, your physician may recommend a stress treadmill test before you start your walking program, just as he would recommend before you start any exercise program.

If you have certain medical conditions, you may have to modify the diet. Patients with severe kidney disease need to be very specific in terms of what they may eat, and they may not do well on this kind of diet. This diet is not for Type I diabetics (lean diabetics who get their diabetes before the age of twenty-five).

If you are on medications, you must discuss this diet with your physician—to find out if this diet will interfere with the efficacy of those medications. You should also discuss when you will need to come back to see your physician again, so that your physician can reduce your medications. One of the great side benefits of this diet is that you will need fewer drugs.

Typically, a person with Type II Diabetes—(obese individuals and those whose onset of diabetes begins after age forty) will start to notice falling glucose levels in just a few days. This may require a reduction in medication.

Patients with hypertension will notice a decrease in their blood pressure in five to seven days—which may require a reduction in their antihypertensive medications. Those persons with high lipids will notice a fall in their cholesterol in about one month.

Your medical condition and the number of different medications you are taking will determine how often you should see your physician. I usually recommend a visit one week after starting the diet and a second visit after one month on the diet.

Before starting the diet, you should have a blood test, and that should be after fasting from the night before the test. *Do not eat after dinner the night of the blood test, except for medications, which should be taken with water only.* The medications can also be taken in the morning with water. This same fasting blood test should be repeated one month after starting the diet.[1]

It is rare for there to be any kind of negative effect from the diet on blood tests. Any abnormal result should be worked up fully by your doctor. Most people see a rapid and marked improvement in glucose and lipids on this diet.

Check with your physician to make sure that you can take all of the vitamins and mineral supplements which I recommend. This is not an all or nothing situation—there are specific situations where one or two of the supplements are not appropriate. You should not take the supplements your doctor tells you are contraindicated for you, but only take the ones that your doctor says are good for you.

The bottom line: check with your doctor before you make any radical change in your diet or exercise.

The Truth About Supplements

Our food today is so processed and adulterated that it is virtually impossible to get all the vitamins and nutrients we need without some sort of supplementation. I'd like to recommend for you the following types of supplementation to accompany the *18% Solution*, so that you get all your nutrition needs met.

---

1.   Depending on your medical condition, you may need to repeat the blood test sooner; ask your physician. The blood test should include: electrolytes; kidney function tests; urinalysis; uric acid, glucose, hemoglobin A1C, urine for microalbumin (for diabetics); calcium, INR (if on Coumadin); liver function; TSH; total cholesterol, HDL, LDL, and triglycerides; CBC, and ferritin.

First, I want you to take one multi-vitamin everyday. You don't have to go to the health food store and get something complicated or expensive—a multi-vitamin like Centrum or One a Day Multi-Vitamin is fine.

Next, I want you to take one baby aspirin per day. Baby aspirin has been proven to reduce strokes and heart attacks. It makes sense for all adults over forty-five to begin taking one baby aspirin per day.

Next, I want you to take three 500 mg. calcium carbonate pills daily with meals. Many people do not consume enough dairy products on the diet, and this supplement will help you avoid calcium deprivation.

Finally, women who are menstruating ought to take one iron pill daily, to maintain a proper level of iron.

This is all the supplementation you need in order to remain healthy! I know that whenever you walk into a health food store, you are probably overwhelmed, as I am, by the astonishing choices that the store offers. Don't worry about it. If you're following the *18% Solution*, you don't really require any of these additional things in order to keep your weight down and your health vibrant.

Condiments

While following the *18% Solution*, you'll want to avoid salt, sugar, oil (including olive oil!) mayonnaise, and ketchup, because all promote weight retention and/or contain unhealthy levels of fat. Salt is treacherous for dieters, so you'll want to work hard to avoid it.

Any fresh spice is fine, and you may use all you like of the following condiments that come in jars: pepper (black or white); garlic (powder only); onion (powder only); mustard; curry; parsley; paprika, and white horseradish.

Cheat to Win!

In an ideal world, once we understand the importance of something, we follow the rules precisely and do things exactly right. In the real world, though, sometimes we do the wrong thing anyway. When it comes to dieting, I realize from my own personal experience and my work with my patients at UCLA that we are always going to have that inner voice urging us to do something mischievous.

This is a long way of saying that everybody cheats on their diets. So it's much more preferable to have a "controlled" form of cheat than an uncontrolled one.

A person on any restricted eating plan will feel deprived. There will always be that inner urge to rebel and cheat. It is far better to build that cheating into the eating plan, so that we can avoid the explosion of uncontrolled cheating down the road.

On the *18% Solution*, you are entitled to a "controlled cheat" once a month after the first month, as you choose. You don't have to have a controlled cheat every month—but you can if you want to. It's not okay to save up your controlled cheats from month to month—and then give yourself a vacation from the diet! That's not permitted on the *18% Solution*! Instead, it's best to pick out a special day, such as a holiday, birthday, anniversary, or restaurant meal as the right time for the controlled cheat.

On your controlled cheat, you can have anything you want from Menu Plan Phase III Stage L, regardless of what stage you are on at the time. Keep in mind that even with a controlled cheat, there will be weight gain.

An individual may gain as much as three to five pounds from that controlled cheat, and that weight may linger for up to five days. Such a relatively small gain may be worth it, so that you don't get into real trouble and blow the plan completely. Sometimes people feel that if you don't do it perfectly, it's blown, which leads to despair. It's only when people feel a sense of despair that they lose the discipline for their diet, give up, and end up shockingly overweight.

Let's talk for a moment about uncontrolled cheats—those that just happen, that are not planned out. If you can turn an uncontrolled cheat into a controlled one, then by all means do so.

If you sense that you are about to embark on an uncontrolled cheat, then try the following strategies. Stuff yourself with permitted foods, such as fruits and vegetables. If that doesn't work, then try hard-boiled eggs. It's awfully hard to eat a whole lot of hard-boiled eggs. If that also fails, then use Phase III Stage L. Whatever you do, don't heed the voice that says, "Since you've cheated a little bit, you might as well give up completely and eat a ton of forbidden foods." The more you cheat, the harder it becomes to get back on the plan.

No matter how much you cheated, and no matter what you ate, get back on the plan immediately. The longer you procrastinate, the more damage you do—and the harder it is to find the resolve to get back on the plan. The next time you eat, eat exactly as you would have had you not slipped.

Please be aware that I'm not giving you license to go off on uncontrolled cheats! If it happens, we have to get back on the plan. It's not something to be encouraged, but if it does happen, let's deal with it the right way. If you have been cheating and go off the plan for a few days, and you have gained more than ten pounds, it is best to go back one stage for a week or two. This will get you back to where you were prior to the cheat. If you have been cheating more than that, it would be best to go back to Stage B for a short while. The main thing is not to despair, and not to quit. There's no shame in falling down. The only shame is in choosing not to get back up.

What To Tell Those Around You

Dear Loved One,

"I have chosen to do the *18% Solution*, a plan that promotes healthy living, wellness, and fitness. It's a very carefully structured plan, with specific and detailed eating and exercise requirements. It's a no starch, low fat diet. In order for me to achieve success on this plan, I have to adhere to it exactly. There is no room whatsoever for any deviations.

"In colloquial language, when it comes to the way I am going to eat from here on in, my suggestion to you is this: **BUTT OUT!**

"I know you care about me, and I know you want to help. But please only help me in the ways in which I ask for help. I don't need any unsolicited advice, because I know exactly what to do. Please don't take charge of my diet. Please don't seek to control how, when, or where I eat, and please don't offer me any unsolicited thoughts or guidance about my diet plan. I trust the physician who has created this plan, and I'm going to give it a fair shot.

"If you want to help me, give me space, give me only positive feedback. Tell me how good I look once I lose some weight. Please be sincere, of course.

"You can also help me by removing all foods not on the *18% Solution* from the house. Please remove them even from the best hiding places—otherwise, I'll find them! And if you're going to cook for me, please only cook foods that are on the plan.

"If you really want to help me, the best thing you can do for me—and for yourself—is to join me on the *18% Solution*! If you are not ready to do that, then at least follow the plan when I am eating with you. Please always follow it when we are at home. Please follow it when you are out with me in a restaurant. Please only suggest that we go to restaurants where I can eat—such as steak and seafood restaurants. Please only order foods that I can eat—it's just too tempting to look at all the foods I'm going to be missing for the next little while!

"Please also be available to go with me for walks and hikes—walking is a very important part of the *18% Solution*. When we walk, let's walk at my pace. Remember—I'm the one with the eating problem, not you!

"Again, please don't constantly question me—please don't ask, 'Should you be eating this?' If it doesn't look like I'm losing weight fast enough, that's my business—not yours!

"Remember that I chose to do this on my own, and I'm responsible only to myself. I know that this program will yield great results, but it's going to be difficult for me. There may be times when I fall down, but as long as I get up and continue on, I will eventually reach my goal. This is as long as I continue to go in the right direction. If I go off the diet for a time, it may take me longer to lose the weight, but I will get there, so please have confidence in me.

"But just in case all of this guidance is a little too complicated to remember, when it comes to the way I'm going to be eating from now on, two simple words will do—**BUTT OUT!**"

Protein and "Energy" Bars: If it Looks Like a Candy Bar and it Tastes Like a Candy Bar …

When you're on the *18% Solution*, I want you to studiously avoid any form of protein bar, power bar, health bar, snack bar, or any energy bar of any kind. Those bars seem so healthy—but the reality is that many of them contain the same number of calories and fat as a candy bar (at twice or three times the price!). If you want a candy bar, why not just eat the real thing—and not fool yourself!

One of the problems with the way we live today is the easy accessibility of high fat, high calorie, high sugar foods. At the supermarket, it's just so easy to reach over to the candy counter at the opposite side of the checkout aisle and grab a chocolate bar. This is just not an option for anyone who is serious about losing weight. *There is no place in the 18% Solution for any form of highly processed, high calorie bars.*

These bars claim to be "meal replacements," but I've never met anyone who ate one protein bar and felt full enough to skip a meal. We have to see these bars for what they really are—highly unhealthy snacks marketed to people who want to lose weight. Just because they sell them in the gym, the health food store, or the drug store does not mean that they are healthy for you. Keep in mind that many drug stores also sell cigarettes!

Instant Meal = Instant Weight Gain

Protein bars are not the only offenders when it comes to high calorie, high fat foods. Most "instant meals" really mean nothing more than instant weight gain for most dieters. For example, instant soup *seems* like such a good idea. It's easy to eat—you just stick the package in the microwave, and you have instant, healthy soup. Here's why you must avoid them:

We're looking at 500 to 600 calories just from that one little bowl of soup, not to mention the incredibly high level of salt it contains. Salt promotes both water retention and hypertension. If it's instant soup, if it's a protein bar, or if it's any other kind of processed food, it's not going to help you lose weight on the *18% Solution*.

Just For Vegetarians

The *18% Solution* absolutely works for vegetarians, many of whom ask, "If I eat so healthy, why am I so overweight?" Contrary to popular belief, "vegetarian" doesn't always equal "healthiest choice." The vegetarian diet, for whatever benefits it may offer, does not in automatically promote weight loss. Let me show you why.

First, many vegetarians cook their vegetables in oil, which is a high calorie food. Coconut oil in particular is absolute poison, due to the highly unhealthy level of trans-fats it contains. Many vegetarians drink soy milk instead of whole milk. Unfortunately, soy milk has a five to seven percent fat content, compared with four percent in whole milk, and obviously lower percentages in skim milk or 1% milk.

Say Nuts to Nuts! (And seeds, avocados, and olives, too!)

Nuts, another favorite choice of vegetarians, are high in oil and fat. Tofu, that staple of vegetarians, also contains five to seven percent of fat by content. The veggie diet also contains lots of starch, which promotes weight retention. So just because you are not eating meat doesn't mean that you are on a diet that is particularly conducive to losing weight or even maintaining weight. You can do the *18% Solution* with low-fat tofu and low-fat soy milk and still get all the protein you need.

Nuts and seeds are good sources of protein, as are avocados and olives. And yet all of these foods are very high in fat. Avocados and olives are over 20% fat by content—and they're not very filling. Nuts and seeds are easy to eat—and therefore we tend to eat a lot of them at any one sitting, especially if we are distracted by television, a book, conversation, or traffic, if we are eating behind the wheel. So nuts, seeds, avocadoes, and olives are all verboten on the *18% Solution*. Keep in mind that a handful of nuts—100 grams or approximately four ounces—contains about 900 calories—and nobody eats just a handful! If the nuts are salted, the situation is worse, because salt promotes fluid retention and hypertension, as we mentioned earlier. So that's why I say nuts to nuts!

A typical medium-sized package of trail mix may contain as much as nine servings of 190 calories per serving. Eating the entire package—not hard to do if we're bored or watching TV (or both)—means that we've just taken in 1,710 theoretically "healthy" calories. But there's nothing healthy about consuming that caloric load in a relatively short period of time, especially when many adults need about that many calories *per day*.

Another illustration of the same point: the other day, I came upon a so-called "diet cookie" in the store. The label promised, in big print, that the cookie only had 100 calories. That looked great, until I looked closer, and discovered that the small print gave away the bad news. The cookie contained 100 calories … per serving! And the cookie contained *four servings!* That was a 400-calorie cookie, rich in diet-smashing salt and starch, just waiting to ensnare the innocent dieter!

In short, just because something is marketed with a health-promoting image doesn't mean it works on the *18% Solution*.

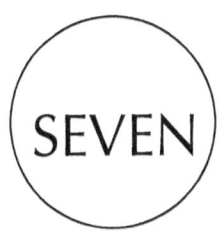

SEVEN

I'VE GOT NO BEEF WITH BEEF!

A million myths surround the issues of eating, weight loss and health. One of the most commonly held beliefs in American society today is that beef is bad for you—that it increases your likelihood of developing heart disease, arteriosclerosis, and a host of other fatal illnesses.

As a UCLA endocrinologist who has thoroughly researched the matter, I'm here to assert that nothing could be further from the truth.

When it comes to cholesterol and weight loss, *there is absolutely no significant or meaningful difference when it comes to eating beef, chicken, or fish.* Many people have given up beef and have turned to eating fish because they believe it is healthier. Meat, chicken, and fish will all deliver the same benefits in terms of diet—and you can eat all the beef you like on this diet, because it will not affect your cholesterol or weight loss in any meaningful way. Raw beef is only fourteen percent fat, versus fifteen percent fat for chicken thighs. The difference is negligible!

The key is to prepare meat in a healthy manner that promotes weight loss. Here's how:

Meats are only to be broiled or barbequed on the *18% Solution*. When you cook this way, much of the fat drips away from the meat. If food is cooked through baking or sautéing, then the food is sitting in the fat while it is being cooked. The meat then absorbs the fat—and so will you. This adds unnecessary calories as well as unnecessary fat to the meat you eat. Non-broiled or non-barbequed meats are not permitted, because they are not a wise nutritional choice.

Make no bones about it: bones are not permitted on meat while it is being barbequed or broiled. The highest fat content of meat is around the bones and inside the marrow of the bones. When the bones are cooked with the meat, it is impossible to keep fat from seeping into the meat. Also, it is so tempting for many of us to gnaw at the bones after they are cooked—which means that we are eating the most fattening part of the meat.

Even during barbequing or broiling, some of the fat will dissolve into the meat. When the meat is eaten, it then contains fat dissolved into it, raising the caloric content and fat content of the meat. This fat is no longer visible after it is cooked, and so it cannot be cut off. Eating meat that is broiled without cutting off the fat before broiling or barbequing is not a healthy choice.

Remove the skin before you broil or barbeque. One of the highest fat deposits of meat is under the skin. When meat is broiled or barbequed, this fat dissolves into the meat. This then raises the fat content of the meat—even if the skin content is removed after cooking and before eating. We're talking extra calories and extra fat—which makes taking weight off harder. This is also, unfortunately a great way to raise cholesterol. So don't barbeque or broil with the skin still on the meat.

Above all, avoid canned meat, marinated meat, and sauces. These are real culprits for dieters, because they are often rich in salt and fat. And you've got to avoid ground meat, deli meat, hamburgers, hot dogs, sausage, and kabobs of all kinds. They're all full of salt and have high fat contents. Packaged meat today contains bristle, bones, fat, and other highly unappetizing parts of the animal. You don't want that in your body, and you certainly don't want to eat that on your diet.

Other meats to avoid: lamb, pork, and duck, because they are high in fat. Turkey and veal are fine.

Beef gets a bad rap not because it's unhealthy. Beef is *fine*. It's the way it is processesed, cooked and served that causes trouble for dieters, and for anyone concerned with his or her health. Again, I've got no beef with beef … as long as you buy it, prepare it, and serve it the right way.

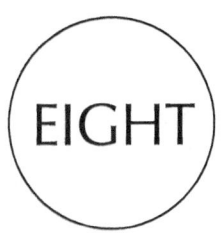

EIGHT

EATING OUT ... WITHOUT SABOTAGING YOUR SUCCESS

When was the last time you went an entire week eating only home-cooked meals?

It's a fact of life in American society that we eat out constantly, and many of us eat out multiple times each week. As you've seen, the 18% Solution is all about vigilance over what you eat, when, how much, and in what manner. So the question naturally arises: how do you reconcile the requirements of the program with the fact that our lifestyles today practically demand that we eat many if not most of our meals away from home?

The good news is that it's possible to keep to the 18% Solution while eating most—or even all—of our meals away from home. It requires a combination of creativity, advance planning, and commitment to the program, but *it can be done.* In this chapter, we'll discuss eating out in social settings, business meals, eating while traveling, and eating at the homes of family and friends ... without sabotaging your success in the 18% Solution program, and without bruising your hosts' feelings!

As you've seen, the 18% Solution is not meant to last a week, a month, or even a year. This is no "quick fix" fad diet! Instead, it is my hope, and my intention, that you will desire to follow the 18% Solution for the rest of your life. My plan is meant as a lifelong approach to food and the question of how to nourish ourselves in a society and culture that practically promotes overeating and even obesity. As we've seen, eating out regularly is a fact of life for most if not all of us, so we need to find a way to reconcile that fact with maintenance of our own personal health goals. Planning ahead and making smart choices is the key.

You will invariably be confronted with all kinds of challenges to maintaining your commitment to the 18% Solution. You must be firm in your resolve not to deviate, no matter what the circumstances! It does take creativity, a special effort, and sometimes even a little bit of assertiveness. Whether it's a social evening out, a business meal, eating out while traveling, a meal at the home of family and friends—you can still remain faithful to your overall goals.

The 18% Solution is not about withdrawing from society so that you can control to the *nth* degree what you eat and when. Rather, it is about finding new ways to enjoy the company of your partner, your spouse, your family, your friends, your relatives, and your business associates. When you travel, you'll be able to conduct your business as before and take in new sights and experiences as well—without losing your focus on the goal of maintaining the 18% Solution. You now have a new goal in life—to satisfy your hunger regularly without sabotaging your success.

Many of us who love food and proudly wear the title of gastronome or gourmet will often plan trips to cities where we can find the finest restaurants, the greatest possible "foodie" experiences, or simply a meal that provides great value for the money. The good news is that you can still travel the world, see the sights, and enjoy a fascinating social life while taking in some of those great restaurants without deviating from your commitment to the 18% Solution. Enjoy your life, plan ahead, don't let yourself get hungry, make good choices, and I guarantee that you will succeed.

Let's now talk about how we implement the 18% Solution "on the road." Let's start with breakfast. Breakfast is generally a relatively simple meal. Of course, it's the key to starting your day right, and under certain circumstances, getting the right kind of breakfast can be a challenge. If you frequent a coffee shop that offers melon, berries, or bananas, you're all set. Yet if your pattern is to stop in at a coffee house or fast food restaurant, then we've got some work to do.

It's unlikely that you'll find fresh fruit in these establishments. So you can still go to them, as long as you plan ahead by sticking one or two grapefruits in your bag or briefcase to enjoy with your coffee. You can continue to enjoy your ritual of enjoying your favorite java, reading the newspaper at the coffee place, or bonding with a friend over breakfast. Now, though, you'll be starting your day the right way, feeling satisfied and energized, and feeling proud of yourself because you've had one more meal that takes you closer to your goal weight … or keeps you there.

It's important to remember that you cannot eat any of the foods that are not on the 18% Solution when you go out for breakfast, regardless of what your companions are having, and regardless of how innocent and harmless that bagel or croissant looks. Keep in mind that those menu staples are not for you! You've found a plan that works for you, and all you have to do now is stick to it … for dear life!

There's certainly a physical reward for you by avoiding the standard breakfast fare of bagels, croissants, muffins, and so on. You're either maintaining your path toward the slender new you you desire, or you are maintaining your dream weight. I also want you to recognize the fact that there is an emotional reward that you'll feel when you successfully take control of this first meal of the day. When you eat an 18% Solution breakfast, you're on the path to success over the course of your day, and that means that you're on a path toward success over the course of your life. What a great way to start the day! CONGRATULATIONS!!!

Now let's talk about lunch. The key to success remains … planning ahead. On work days, the best approach is to bring food, like melon or grapefruit, from home, or purchase some produce at a market on the way to work. Most quality supermarkets offer wonderful fresh salad bars. Remember to avoid the dressings, nuts, seeds, bacon bits, croutons, and marinated vegetables, which are loaded with oil and salt. The 18% Solution isn't just for the home, especially when we consider just how many meals we eat outside the house. Work your plan even at the supermarket salad bar!

Perhaps you eat lunch in restaurants or coffee shops on an occasional basis or even every day. Where possible, try to select establishments that offer salad bars, or an array of fresh vegetables or fruit. If you're a regular customer, let the manager or maitre d' know how he or she can best accommodate you. They will enjoy meeting your special needs every bit as much as you will enjoy the fact that they are looking out for your best interests. If you're going to a new restaurant, study the menu even before you sit down. Ask the hostess if the restaurant will be able to meet your needs. If not, working your plan is a lot more important than your convenience, so don't hesitate to smile, leave, and find another restaurant nearby. Many restaurants will gladly accommodate you if you ask and are assertive, especially if you are a regular customer.

If the restaurant *can* work with your 18% Solution requirements, stay and order a fruit appetizer and then a salad. If you finish your salad and you're still hungry, eat a second one! Always make sure you leave the restaurant feeling satisfied and satiated, so that you don't end up bingeing later!

Always emphasize to your server your specific dietary needs when you order. Confirm with your waiter or waitress exactly how the food will be prepared. Some servers might humor you and tell you they will follow your dietary requests, and then fail to follow through. You do not have to accept food that is not made in accordance with the requests to which your server has agreed. Again, it takes a little bit of assertiveness, but the payoff for your "sticking to your guns" will be fantastic, in terms of your own continued weight loss and the good feelings you'll have about yourself because you have stayed true to your commitment.

It's best to frequent a few restaurants often, so they come to know you and your requests. When you become a frequent customer, they will make sure to accommodate your special desires without a hassle. Steakhouses and fish restaurants are your best choices for "homes away from home." Be emphatic—you will not accept marinated food or food cooked in sauces or with dressings. If the restaurant serves small portions—often the case in upscale restaurants—don't stay hungry. If after you finish your first main course you are still hungry, don't hesitate to order a second main course! Keep in mind that it's a lot cheaper to order a second main course than to leave yourself hungry ... and trigger an expensive—both in dollars and calories—binge later on.

While waiting for your order to arrive, avoid the bread. While other people are having an appetizer or soup, you can have fruit if it is available, or a salad without dressing. Remember always to order salad with no dressing instead of the side dishes with the main course. You don't even want the side dishes on your plate—the temptation can be too overpowering! If the others in your party order dessert, you can order fruit. If you're with friends, you'll probably want to linger after dessert for twenty minutes or half an hour. So order a beverage while you sit around and talk. If others are ordering wine or liqueurs, you can order Perrier or decaffeinated coffee or tea. There's no reason at all to feel deprived during your dining out experience. Focus on all the foods you *can* enjoy, not the ones you can't have. Focus on the ambiance, and the good time you are having with your spouse, date, partner, or friends. If you are still hungry when you come home, enjoy some fruit ... until those hunger pangs diminish.

What happens if you find yourself in a Chinese restaurant, a pizza place, or a fast food establishment? These are clearly not good choices for your plan, and you should avoid them whenever possible. Yet sometimes these places are inevitable, especially if you are with a group from work or on the road. My strong suggestion here is to have a soda or other beverage with everyone, so that you can enjoy the social aspects of the experience. Don't eat until you get home, though, or eat when you can get to a supermarket and buy plenty of fresh produce that is good for you. It's even better to eat some food before you meet the gang at the Chinese restaurant or fast food outlet, so you are not hungry and miserable watching everyone else enjoy all that mouth-watering food. You may even want to make a habit of stocking a few apples in your car or briefcase. Apples are not especially perishable and will do the trick of taking the edge off your hunger until you find an eating situation that works for you.

The best places to eat out are fish restaurants, steakhouses, and upscale American and European style restaurants that are in the business of pleasing customers with far more finicky requests than ours. Again, there's almost nothing for us to eat in a fast food restaurant, a pizza shop or a Chinese restaurant, even though we used to enjoy those kinds of meals. We're going to have give up some of our favorite restaurants in order to reach our goals. Anything worth achieving requires a little bit of self-sacrifice, and that's certainly true when it comes to losing weight, keeping that weight off, and improving the quality of our health and our lives. That's all that the 18% Solution suggests about dining out.

Now let's talk about eating at home. If you keep focused on your goals of living a long, healthy life, and you are "eating to live," eating in your own home, even if you have guests over, will not present a problem, since you get to choose the menu. The easiest thing to do is to plan at least part of the menu in terms of the 18% Solution. You're certainly free to prepare other "non-approved" foods for your guests. That depends on the nature of the function and whom you have invited.

Keep in mind that you can be very creative with fresh fruit, fresh vegetables, and lean meat. You can combine these elements to make great salads and other dishes. Just remember not to use salt, oil, or mayonnaise, and you can still serve the salads with many different dressings, in accordance with the 18% Solution. Also keep in mind that today, just about everybody is watching his or her weight! So your guests will almost certainly thank you for your thoughtfulness in providing healthy, delicious food for them.

You can serve these foods at dinner parties both elegant or informal. Hors d'oeuvres can include meats in bite-size pieces arranged on platters, with mustard or horseradish on the side. At elegant functions, you can have carving stations serving turkey or prime rib. Desserts can include exotic fruits like raspberries, mango, and papaya. At more informal gatherings, barbecue and salad bars should pose no problem for you. If you find that you must serve other foods that are not on the 18% Solution, remember to eat only foods that are permissible for you! No cheating—you can't even taste the other food if you're serious about weight loss.

If you're going to eat out, plan ahead. If you know where you are going to have lunch, research the kind of food the restaurant serves and determine in advance how accommodating they might be to your requirements. If you're going to eat at home, you get to plan the menu. But what if you're going to someone else's home for a meal?

Remember the foods on the 18% Solution are extremely easy to obtain and prepare. So your host or hostess is not likely to feel imposed upon by your request. Anyone who cares about you will be more than happy to buy a "ready pack" bag of salad in a supermarket and add rice vinegar, or purchase a filet of beef or fish from the supermarket or from a butcher to broil or barbecue. Remember, you cannot have beef, chicken, or fish that has been marinated or sprayed with spice for "flavor." You cannot have chicken or turkey cooked with the skin, or in sauces, even if they are removed later.

Other 18% Solution "no-nos" include dark meat chicken, or anything breaded or fried. Practically everybody is on a diet of some sort these days, so it won't come as a shock for your host or hostess if you courteously set forth your food needs with enough time in advance to allow for proper shopping and preparation. And who knows? Maybe your host or hostess could stand dropping a few pounds, too … and maybe they'll want to hear all about the 18% Solution from you! That's especially true if you've been on the program for a while, and the evidence of your weight loss is there for all to see in the form of your attractive new shape and your positive attitude.

Enjoying the meal in a friend's home will be a pleasant and successful experience on the 18% Solution … as long as you plan ahead. Remember that if people invite you to eat at their house, they are your friends, and they want the best for you. They want you to succeed on your diet plan. Keep in mind, though, that a little bit of courtesy on your part goes a long way. Most people hosting dinner parties are tense as the big day approaches and are almost certainly worried about last minute details. Springing special requests on a host at the time of the party, or even the same day, is truly unfair and may cause resentment. Your hosts will feel hurt if they have put a lot of time, energy, creativity, and love into a menu, and at the last minute you tell them you will not eat the food that they have so joyously prepared. You can avoid this discomfort all around by notifying your host with as much advance notice as possible about your special dietary needs.

In sum, the 18% Solution is flexible enough to meet your needs wherever you travel and whenever you eat outside your home. A little forethought will lead to a lot of weight loss ... and that's what it's all about!

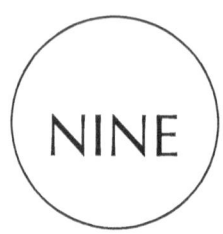

NINE

WHY DO YOU WANT TO LOSE WEIGHT, AND WHAT HOLDS YOU BACK?YOU

In my UCLA practice, I ask my patients to dig deeply into their psyches to discover exactly why they want to lose weight. The answers they give me: to feel better, to be healthier, to look better, and to feel better about themselves. These are very appropriate motivators for weight loss that people commonly recognize in themselves. So if people know *why* they want to lose weight and they know *how* to lose weight (eat in a healthier fashion and exercise more), then why is it so hard for them to succeed in their weight loss and then to keep that weight off?

In this chapter, I'd like to discuss with you some of the barriers that exist to accomplishing the goal of losing weight. I believe there are two basic categories—physiological barriers and psychological barriers. The physiological barriers are fairly straightforward. Here's a list of the most common ones:

- not knowing how bad certain foods are for us.

- not understanding the correct amount to eat for our metabolic needs.

- not doing enough exercise.

These physiological barriers are relatively easy to deal with, in comparison to the psychological ones, in that they only require education and a strong will. Once we understand the danger to a foodaholic of the single french fry, to give a somewhat dramatic example, we know what we must do, and what we must avoid doing. Thus these barriers can be overcome.

This leaves the psychological barriers, which are truly challenging to deal with. Foodaholics don't eat because they are physiologically hungry. They eat because of psychological needs. You may recognize this from personal experience. How many times have you said that you were so full that you could not eat another thing, and yet you managed to polish off a bag of candy, a container of ice cream, or a package of cookies? I'm just as guilty—keep in mind that I created this 18% Solution primarily for myself before I even thought about sharing it with friends and patients!

When we eat in an out-of-control manner, we are doing so not because we need energy, but to give ourselves pleasure and to treat ourselves. We need to demonstrate the fact that we are in control. A foodaholic might eat a donut and say to himself, "No one's gonna tell me what to eat! No one's gonna boss me around, not my doctors, not my wife, not my kids, not my friends!" That demonstrates control, although not in a healthy way! We also eat in an out-of-control manner to avoid unpleasant thoughts. We will eat to show that we are not different from those around us. If everyone else is enjoying pasta at the dinner table, we don't want to be the only one eating salad! If they're at the game drinking beer and eating potato chips, we want to fit in—we don't want to be sitting there drinking bottled water and eating celery sticks!

Let's take a look at some of the psychological components of the resistance we have toward eating right.

Need for reward.

Perhaps you've been working on a project for weeks. You've dedicated countless hours to it, on top of your regular responsibilities. The project is finished, but all you get is a cursory thank you. Everyone else is ready to move on ... except you. You, on the other hand, feel that you should have received more recognition and appreciation in honor of having completed such a monumental task. Yet no one gave you a party ... so you treat yourself to a party of your own. You will eat ice cream, or cake, or french-fries, or quarter-pounders—whatever your favorite "naughty" food may be. Of course, no one else is invited to this party, and the eating will generally take place in the privacy of your own kitchen, when no one else is around, often late at night, or even in your automobile. Anyplace where no one else knows just how much (or how quickly!) you are eating.

The worse we feel emotionally, the less we have to do in order to believe we deserve a special reward, and that reward often takes the form of a binge. In many cases, individuals feel they deserve a few donuts simply for getting out of bed in the morning or for getting dressed. The more weight we gain, the lower our self-esteem, the more parties we deserve, and so we eat more and gain more weight on this vicious cycle. Clearly, rewarding ourselves through food is a self-destructive act.

Rewarding unpleasant jobs.

Another psychological reason for eating is to avoid unpleasant tasks. Anything from taking out the garbage to preparing our taxes can trigger a "hunger message"—instead of doing what we need to do, we find comfort in the refrigerator or freezer. We can delay almost any unpleasant task by eating. As silly as it sounds, we can even eat to delay starting a diet! The more negative our attitude about things, the more tasks we find unpleasant, the more things we therefore wish to delay. So the more unpleasant we find life, the more we want to eat.

Avoiding unpleasant thoughts.

We may not even want to *think* about our finances, let alone open that Visa bill or start working on our taxes. So we delay by eating. We might also not want to think about a lot of other important things—our relationships, our careers, health, weight, and so on. When we are instead concentrating on how much "naughty" stuff we will eat, when, and how, we are diverting our minds from the unpleasant thoughts we would rather not face. An added "fringe benefit," if you can call it that, of binge eating, is that after we eat out of control we are so busy beating ourselves up emotionally, and then feeling so sorry for ourselves, that we definitely don't have the time or energy to focus on the other, underlying unpleasant thoughts.

That soothing, suckling sensation.

We eat also because the need for the chewing and suckling sensation satisfies our need to soothe ourselves. It doesn't matter what we chew in order to experience that soothing feeling. Generally, we chew high calorie foods when we look for relief through eating.

Demonstrating control.

Another psychological reason for eating in an out-of-control manner is to demonstrate that we are actually in control of what, when, and how much we eat. "You can't tell me not to have a whole container of ice cream!" we think, in a somewhat childish manner. "I'll show you I can eat as much as I want, whenever I want!" We are trying to show the outside world we are in control. Instead, we are actually sending the world the opposite message—that we are totally out of control of our eating. So by seeking to demonstrate control to ourselves and the world, we are actually demonstrating just how out of control we truly are.

Being foodaholics.

Many of us eat because we are foodaholics or food addicts. Those of us who "cop to" this label are just as addicted to food as the drug addict is to drugs, the alcoholic to alcohol, the gambler to gambling, and a smoker to lighting up. The foodaholic does not eat because he is hungry from a metabolic perspective, but because he has an addictive craving that must be assuaged. The foodaholic does not care how full he is, or even what he's eating, once he begins to give into his craving. Instead, he will gorge himself and often eat until he either runs out of food or time for eating.

"It's not fair!"

"It's not fair that everyone else can eat that!" If everyone else can eat it, we rationalize to ourselves that we should be able to eat it, too. Thus we show ourselves that we are not different from other people. Few of us want to stand out, and by telling ourselves or others that we are different because we cannot eat certain foods, we fear that we are going to "stick out from the crowd" in a psychologically or socially unpleasant way. Of course, few people can "get away" with eating large amounts of high fat, high cholesterol, high salt, high starch foods for long. The habit catches up with us in our waistline, and the habit also catches up with us in terms of the physical illnesses associated with overeating that are discussed elsewhere in this book. Don't compare yourself to that rare skinny friend or relative who can eat an ice cream sundae or brownie and not gain weight. If you can't eat a certain food without gaining weight, join the crowd!

Putting It All Together.

Many of my patients have heard me discuss this list of psychological barriers to weight loss, and their reaction has been to throw up their hands and to feel that overeating is a compulsion beyond their ability to halt. They often feel there is nothing they can do to overcome their "foodaholic" tendencies. I always urge them—and you—not to give up! The 18% Solution is a plan that will work for you to overcome both the physiological and psychological barriers to weight loss. The operative word here is "plan." This truly is a plan that will work, and this plan has a number of components. When you take all of the components together—the phases and stages, the permitted and forbidden foods, the approaches to eating at home, in restaurants, and in homes of others, the plan will work for you, as it has for countless others. Keep in mind that working one component by itself will not get the job done. You're going to need the "whole enchilada!" Keep in mind also that you've been functioning and thinking one particular way about eating for years and years, so it's going to take a long time before all of your old eating habits are replaced with healthier ones. The plan I have outlined for you in this book—the 18% Solution—will address all the psychological needs and deal with them in a positive way, instead of the negative way it may have been handled in your life up to the present moment. So let's take a look at ways to cope with the psychological barriers to weight loss.

Break the vicious cycle.

Begin to break your vicious cycle by doing something positive in your life. This will be good for you and it will make you feel good about yourself. You're already doing it, by having developed a consciousness about your current approach to eating, but now it's time to formalize your commitment to yourself. One way to demonstrate that commitment is to go out for a leisurely twenty-minute walk. I want you to walk for twenty minutes without stopping. You can walk on the street, in a park, on a track, at a shopping mall, or on a treadmill. Whatever your choice, it should be flat and cool where you walk. This easy activity is available to anyone, and it will start your positive cycle. Once you have accomplished your first twenty-minute walk, you'll feel like a winner. Your self-esteem will rise. You'll realize that you are doing something for yourself that is good for you. You'll see that there is no reason to do something counterproductive and injurious to yourself, like eating something fattening. Once you put out the effort of twenty minutes to walk, you will suddenly realize what a waste of effort it is to counteract that positive act by eating something unhealthy in twenty seconds.

Reward yourself.

You *do* deserve a reward. You should be allowed to eat as much as you want. The reward for your commitment to the 18% Solution is eating food and chewing, and it really doesn't matter what the healthy food you choose might be. Feel free to choose a food such as an exotic fruit—a treat and reward, but not a high calorie splurge. If you want a food reward, and there's no reason not to give yourself one, then treat yourself with luxurious food consistent with the plan, such as a meal of papaya, endive salad, filet mignon, and raspberries for dessert. That sounds like a great meal, don't you agree? Or choose something crunchy that you can chew, such as a carrot, celery, or a cucumber if you just want something to chew on.

Rewards do not always have to be foods. You can also reward yourself by buying yourself a new book, or scarf, or a CD. Treat yourself by going to a museum, a movie, or a show. Be specific in reminding yourself that this reward is for a certain accomplishment or milestone on your eating plan.

You can also have a reward of doing something healthy for yourself. Walking can be looked upon as a treat. It is time by yourself, away from the office, the phones and e-mail, time to think, look at scenery, or listen to music. This is a reward with benefits only—no drawbacks whatsoever!

Learn to constructively avoid unpleasant jobs.

Alas, there will always be unpleasant tasks in our lives. We'll instinctively want to find ways to avoid doing them. The main thing is not to cause ourselves harm when we avoid those unpleasant tasks, be it raking the leaves, shoveling snow, or doing those taxes. For example, if you feel the urge to procrastinate through eating, don't beat yourself up! Give in! Just make sure that whatever you eat is something permissible on the 18% Solution. Keep in mind that you're not eating because you care about what you're eating—you just want to eat so you don't have to do the thing you don't want to do! If you're going to eat, in other words, just make sure that you don't sabotage your 18% Solution program.

A positive way of avoiding unpleasant thoughts.

If you are strict with your eating plan, you will have fewer unpleasant thoughts that you will want to avoid. This is a wonderful side benefit of the program. You won't have to think about your weight, and you won't feel depressed about failing at trying to control it, because now you are on a path to achieving your ideal weight … and maintaining it forever. Again, if you feel the urge to eat to avoid the unpleasant thoughts that do arise, make sure you're eating something that is on the 18% Solution … since, again, you really don't care what you're eating, anyway! Ultimately, the more weight you lose, the fewer the times that you will feel the urge to eat in order to avoid unpleasant thoughts.

Fulfilling your suckling need.

Don't fight that built-in need for the comfort that suckling—chewing on food—gives you. Instead, go with it. Just remember that the soothing aspect comes from the chewing, not from the high caloric content of the foods. In other words, you can get that same psychological benefit from eating fruit that you can from eating ice cream! Always eat something that is on the 18% Solution, since, once again, it's not about the specific food. It's about the psychological craving that we all have for the comfort that comes from suckling or chewing. Crunchy foods such as apples, pears, carrots, and cucumbers will fulfill your desire to be soothed just as well as things like ice cream, cookies, and other high calorie, high risk foods.

Demonstrate your control!

We want to demonstrate our control by showing that we can eat what we want, when we want, and that we are not "victims" of cravings. Positive control, by contrast, means that other people cannot dictate what we are going to eat, and neither can that "voice in the back of our minds" that urges us to eat that cookie or buy that container of ice cream. If you go to a party, don't be afraid to look different because you're not eating precisely what the host serves. It's not healthy for you. If it's not on the 18% Solution, then be true to yourself … instead of worrying what other people think. When your friends say, "Let's go for pizza," stay in control—go, but stick to diet soda. Enjoy the social aspect of the gathering, but avoid the empty calories and the starch that the 18% Solution helps you avoid. If you go and eat pizza just because your friends do, you're letting them control you. You demonstrate control over yourself by avoiding the "food cues" in that situation that would have you go off the 18% Solution.

Breaking the foodaholic cycle.

Foodaholics do not eat because of true hunger from a metabolic point of view, but because they have an addictive craving. As we have seen, foodaholics do not care how full they are. Once they give in to their craving, they gorge themselves, and as we have seen, often eat until they run out of food or run out of time for eating. Yet foodaholics can break this cycle, just as alcoholics can break the cycle of problem drinking.

Keep in mind that the more you eat of the "bad" foods, the more you want to eat them. The first bite of the bad foods is the most dangerous. You can't eat just one bite! Nobody can! Keep in mind, as they say in Alcoholics Anonymous, when you're run over by a train, it's the engine that causes all the damage, not the caboose! So avoid that first bite, and you won't have to worry about the rest.

The key is to stop eating the bad foods and fill up instead on good foods. It's fruitless (no pun intended) to fight the urge to eat. You will always lose. Just substitute good foods. You really don't care what you eat, as long as you are eating. You are encouraged to eat as much of the good foods as you desire. Food addiction is like any addiction—it is never cured. You are only in remission for the time that you are actively working a program to keep your addiction in abeyance. Even if you lose all the weight you wish and you are at your ideal weight, if you start eating the bad foods again, you will be back on the addiction route to regaining all your weight (and more) again. When it comes to your addiction, you must always be responsible.

Be different.

Most of us eat when, where, and what everyone else is eating, just so that we can fit in and avoid being different. In reality, each of us is unique and different from everyone else on earth. We each have individual eye color, hair texture, hair color, and height. These are physical differences we can do nothing about. We also have different abilities and talents. Some of us are great at sports and others are handy at fixing things. Some of us have an aptitude for science and math, while others love literature and languages. And some of us have the genetic gift of a metabolism that allows us to be lean. Others—most people, myself and probably you have received a metabolism through the genetic process which, if unchecked, will make you overweight.

As with everything else in life, in those areas where we do not have a natural or genetic gift, we can often compensate by working harder. Perhaps you had a friend in school who overcame a weakness in a particular subject by hiring a tutor or studying longer hours than anyone else. A little extra hard work brought substantial rewards. Well, the same is true when it comes to eating—that extra effort can make a big difference. If we recognize that we don't have a natural lean metabolism, we can work extra hard by following the 18% Solution and be successful. Getting into that whiny "It's not fair" mode isn't productive and won't help you lose the weight. Remember, life really isn't fair. So just compensate and try even harder for success. You can make it!

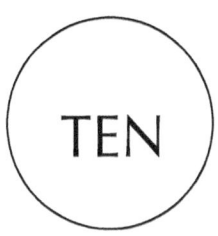

TEN

KEEPING IT OFF ... FOREVER

Many people fear that if they are going to remain "true" to their diet, they'll have to eat "rabbit food" for the rest of their lives! Sound depressingly familiar?

That's not true at all of the 18% Solution, which is much more liberal than many other well-known diets. The intense phase of the 18% Solution lasts only a relatively short period of time. And then there's light at the end of the tunnel—wine, popcorn, breads, many of the delicious foods that most dieters fear they'll never enjoy again.

The 18% Solution teaches you how to get to your ideal weight, and how to keep your weight there. It teaches you how to eat right and how to lose weight through staged advancement of your diet. More important, the 18% Solution teaches you how to continue to eat right and keep the weight off.

There's good news and bad news about the 18% Solution. First the bad news: on this diet, as on any other program, once you lose the weight, if you go back to your old style of eating, you'll gain all your weight back, and perhaps even more. The good news about the 18% Solution is that it teaches you through a succession of stages how to eat right. If you're committed to eating right, you will know what to do in all situations, and you'll be able to do it relatively easily.

If you want to keep your weight off, it will never be possible again to eat things like French fries or deep fried fish. Such things are simply incompatible with maintaining one's ideal weight.

(By the way, no one stays at his or her ideal weight all the time! We vary by a few pounds for many factors. So I recommend to my patients that they actually try to stay a few pounds beneath their ideal weight, to give themselves a little leeway in case a few pounds creep back.)

The good news is that you will be able to have a baked potato or sushi, and you'll find these more healthful choices considerably more satisfying than the "comfort foods" we are leaving behind. You may not be able to enjoy something like apple turnovers, but you will be able to get more pleasure out of a baked apple. And so on. The 18% Solution is here to teach you how to make the best choices, understand why you are making them, and stick to them.

Obviously, before you can maintain your ideal weight, you have to get there! On the 18% Solution, you will advance through the maintenance stages and add foods, as long as you keep losing weight. You'll come to realize that when you add certain other foods, you will no longer lose weight, but in fact start to gain again. The knowledge of what you can eat to keep weight off and what foods will cause weight gain, will be the key information for you to keep at your maintenance weight. In order to keep the weight off for the long term, you need to get to your ideal weight first.

Once you get to your ideal weight, I would like to see you lose at least five more pounds, and that way you've got a little bit of a margin to work with. I suggest to my patients that they eat foods at the highest stage in the 18% Solution that allows them to stay at the "five pounds below ideal weight" level. Weigh yourself at least twice a week to make sure that you are keeping to that ideal place. Once you gain any weight so that you are less than five pounds below your ideal weight, go back to Stage B and stay on it until you return to that blissful "five pounds below ideal" level. At that point, you can go back to your maintenance stage.

If your weight does go above "five pounds below ideal," the important thing is to go back to Stage B at once. Do not allow yourself to be fooled into the belief that since you lost so much weight, more weight will come off by itself. Weight never comes off by itself! This could well be the beginning of the end of your new, svelte body … so don't take that chance!

A common experience of my patients is that once they reach their ideal weight, they begin to rationalize. They start asking themselves questions like, "What's the big difference between a baked potato and hash browns?" Or "What's the big difference between fat-free, sugar-free frozen yogurt on the one hand and ice cream on the other?" The difference … is a lot of calories, and a lot of fat. To eat correctly for the long term, it's important for you to recognize that you have a different metabolism than other people and you'll never be able to eat a "standard American diet." Keep in mind that most people on that "standard American diet" (lots of starch, lots of sugar, lots of fat) are dangerously overweight. Remember that you are not on a diet for a month, six months, or a year, or even three years to lose a certain amount of weight, and then you can eat "whatever." If you're serious about maintaining your weight loss, you can never eat "whatever"! Anytime you have a big meal of "whatever" you are off your eating program, with the disastrous likely consequences ahead.

Keep your mind on the 18% Solution at all times. When you're at a party, you want to be telling yourself "That egg roll looks and smells great, but it's not worth eating it and then gaining four or five pounds." Yes, you will get the urge to cheat, but you need to know how to counter it. You need to practice stuffing yourself on permissible foods. Pile your plate high with raw vegetables and raw fruit. If you luck out and find yourself at a party offering sashimi, pig out on the fish ... but avoid the rice! Play by the rules and the results you desire will be yours.

As we've discussed throughout this book the second component of keeping your weight off for the long term is exercise. Exercise is not optional. It's mandatory, on a daily basis. Many studies have shown that only those individuals who do daily aerobic exercise succeed over the long term with weight maintenance. There are many reasons for this, both metabolic and psychological. I think the most important reason for the importance of exercise is psychological, however. If you spend an hour working hard exercising, it's far less likely that you will find it worthwhile to cheat on your diet. You'll understand that an hour of walking on a treadmill to burn off the calories in one bagel just isn't worth it. You'll find that it's too much work to try to burn off a muffin or a cheesecake. The "magic bullet" for successfully keeping your weight off for the long term ... is daily aerobic exercise.

It's also vital to recognize that you, like so many people (you're not alone!) do not have an accurate hunger mechanism. People like us do not eat only when we are physiologically hungry and need more calories for energy. Your body most likely gives you messages that you *perceive* as hunger, but these are really messages that you need loving, affection, and the sense that you are cared for.

A foodaholic will often go without breakfast and lunch and not feel hungry all day long. That same person will feel hungry for a cookie, or even a box of cookies, however, after having eaten a large six-course meal. So for us, it's not about the energy. It's about the feelings we get when we eat ... especially when we feed ourselves the "comfort foods," those food items that have no place in the 18% Solution. Keeping your weight off for the long term means never eating simply because you're hungry and you see something that looks delicious. Instead, it's about learning to eat by the clock. This means that we eat only at the scheduled eating times, and we force ourselves to eat then, whether we are hungry or not.

This means that we need breakfast, a midmorning snack, lunch, a mid-afternoon snack, dinner, and a bedtime snack. We need to schedule these meals no matter how busy we are and whether we are hungry or not.

Eating by the clock also means eating "by the page." We don't eat what looks delicious or appetizing or what smells good. Instead, we eat only what is on the printed page of the stage of the 18% Solution on which we currently find ourselves. Whether we eat at home or not, we eat only what is on our printed diet sheet.

When you come to think of it, there is never a reason to look at a menu in a restaurant! You need to order exactly what you are permitted to eat on the 18% Solution, not what they have on the menu. Let's say you go into a restaurant and decide you want fish, chicken or meat. So you would ask the waitress, "What kind of filet do you have?" She would then tell you. You then order that meal cooked on the grill, rare or well done, with no spices or sauces. Ask for it served on a plate with no side dishes—not even steamed vegetables. Then ask for some cut up lettuce, cucumbers, carrots, and mushrooms in a big bowl, without dressing, as a replacement for the side dishes with your meat. Then ask, "What kind of fruit do you have?" Have some for an appetizer, and some more for dessert. There's no reason to look at the menu—it can only get you in trouble!

Planning is the key. A good way to accomplish this is to write out a schedule of eating for the next day, each night before you go to bed. You can do it by hand, on a PDA, or on your office computer. The trick is to have it down concretely, where you can see it and live by it. The schedule needs to include the exact time to eat each of these six meals (at a minimum), where you will eat each of those meals, exactly what you will eat for each of those six meals, in accordance with your current stage on the 18% Solution. Most critically, your eating plan should include in detail how you will transport that food to the place where you're going to eat it! For example, if I know I'm going to eat a mango for lunch, I must write down that it is the mango I have in the refrigerator, and I will bring it with me to work. Or if I'm going to have a fruit plate at a business meeting, I must document on my eating plan the individual at the meeting or at the restaurant who will arrange for me to get my fruit plate.

It sounds like a lot of work, and I freely admit that it's harder to remain on the 18% Solution than it is to simply eat whatever looks good, tastes good, and feels good. The problem is the result caused by unrestrained eating. When you stay on the 18% Solution, you lose weight quickly, efficiently, and permanently. When we allow ourselves to return to our old, less disciplined eating habits, we simply won't get the results we desire—a healthy, slim body, great health, and the pride and self-esteem that comes from knowing we have accomplished something extremely important in our lives.

I hope that you will give the 18% Solution a fair try. It has helped many people with severe weight problems to conquer their decades-long struggle to eat right and become—and remain—lean and healthy. I know the program will work for you if you give it a chance. So let's turn now to the diets that are at the core of the program. I'll be with you as you go through the phases ... every step of the way!

THE 18% SOLUTION
GENERAL GUIDELINES

If you have any medical condition, you must check with your physician before starting on this diet.

If you take any medications, pills or injections, whether by prescription or over the counter, you MUST check with your physician and have the dosages of the medications adjusted.

If it is all right with your physician, you should take the following supplements daily.

One Multivitamin daily. (Such as Centrum or One A Day Multivitamin)

One baby aspirin daily.

Three Calcium Carbonate 500 mg each daily (OK if contains additional minerals such as magnesium or Vitamin D.

One Iron supplement daily for women who menstruate. (Such as Ferrous Sulfate)

You must drink at least 64 oz. of liquid per day. (2 quarts or 8–8 oz. glasses—about two liters)

Do not drink any liquid ½ hour before or ½ hour after eating, or while eating any food.

You must eat some fruit every three hours. It can be as little as a quarter of an apple or a quarter of a grapefruit.

You must exercise DAILY as follows:

1st week—Walk one mile per day.

2nd week—Walk one and ¼ miles per day.

3rd week—Walk one and ½ miles per day

4th week—Walk one and ¾ miles per day.

5th week—Walk two miles per day.

6th week—Walk two and ¼ miles per day.

7th week—Walk two and ½ miles per day.

8th week—Walk two and ¾ miles per day.

9th week—Walk three miles per day.

Thereafter walk at least 3 miles per day.

You should see your physician monthly to check your blood pressure and get blood tests.

THE 18% SOLUTION
SEASONINGS

Only the following may be used from jars or cans. **Everything else must be fresh!**

Pepper (black or white)

Garlic (Powder Only)

Onion (Powder Only)

Mustard

Curry

Parsley (Flakes Only)

Paprika

White Horseradish

THE 18% SOLUTION
BEVERAGES

You must drink 64 oz. of water per day. (2 quarts = 8 x 8 oz. glasses)

Bottled or Tap **not carbonated**

Preferably you should not drink within a half an hour of eating

You may not drink Fruit or Vegetable Juice (fresh, canned or frozen)

You may drink diet soda. It is not encouraged. **One can maximum daily.**

You may drink **unsweetened Tea**. Cold or hot. Decaffeinated or Herbal preferred.

Only Diet Snapple or other Diet Tea drinks are permitted.

You may drink coffee. Cold or hot. Decaffeinated or Herbal preferred.

No Sugar, No Whiteners, No Creamers, No Powders,

No Soy Milk, No Half and Half, No Mocha Mix.

You may use Sweet'n Low or Equal or Splenda

You may add up to ½ oz. of non fat milk per cup of coffee

You may not drink Alcoholic Beverages

No wine, no beer, no liquor.

THE 18% SOLUTION
Phase I—III
Stages AA—L
Stage X

THE 18% SOLUTION
Cleansing & Relearning—Phase I (Alternate)
Stage AA

1. All of **One Kind of Fresh Fruit** you want to eat. You must stay on the same fruit the whole time you are on stage AA. The best fruits to choose from are grapefruit, orange, and cantaloupe. (**Fresh Only!!!—Not frozen or canned or dried or juiced or cooked.**) No nuts. No seeds. No cocoanut. No watermelon. No grapes. No bananas.

2. All the **Fresh Raw Vegetables** you want to eat. Unlike fruit, you can have a variety of all of the different kinds of vegetables you desire! Mix them into a salad or eat them by themselves, as you choose. (**Fresh Only!!!—Not frozen or canned or dried or juiced or cooked or micro-waved.**)
   You may put on lemon juice or any kind of vinegar.
   (**No Oil and No Salad Dressing.**) No avocado. No olives.

3. At **one** meal per day all the **Lean, One Kind of Protein** you want to eat from the list below. (**Broiled or BBQ'd, No Sauces, No Bones, No Fat, No Skin.**)

Fish	No Shellfish
Beef	
	No chopped meat
	No ground meat
Veal	
Chicken	White Meat Only
Turkey	White Meat Only
Tuna	White Meat—Water Packed—Low Salt

<u>Sample Menu</u>
Cleansing & Relearning—Phase I (Alternate)
Stage AA

Breakfast

Fruit of the Month

Beverage (½ hour before meal, or ½ hour after meal)

Mid-Morning Snack

Fruit of the Month

Beverage (½ hour before meal, or ½ hour after meal)

Lunch

Salad

Fruit of the Month

Beverage (½ hour before meal, or ½ hour after meal)

Mid-Afternoon Snack

Fruit of the Month

Beverage (½ hour before meal, or ½ hour after meal)

Dinner

Fruit of the Month

Salad

Meat, Chicken, or Fish

Fruit of the Month

Beverage (½ hour before meal, or ½ hour after meal)

Evening Snack

Fruit of the Month

Diet Tips
Cleansing & Relearning—Phase I (Alternate)
Stage AA

1. The most filling fruit is a grapefruit. An orange is the next most filling. After that come the melons.

2. A good way to give the filet of chicken flavor is to marinate the chicken in vinegar, water, mustard, white horseradish, onion, and garlic, and then broil or BBQ.

3. It is O.K. to sprinkle Sweet 'n Low on grapefruit, strawberries or other fruit.

THE 18% SOLUTION
Cleansing & Relearning—Phase I
Stage A

1.   All of **One Kind of Fresh Fruit** you want to eat. You may change your selection each morning, but you've got to stick with one particular fruit each day. If you have an orange, stick to oranges. The next day, you can choose a different fruit, say, apples ... but stick to apples for that whole day. (**Fresh Only!!!—Not frozen or canned or dried or juiced or cooked.**) No nuts. No seeds. No cocoanut. No watermelon. No grapes. No bananas.

2.   All the **Fresh Raw Vegetables** you want to eat. You can have all of the different kind of vegetables you desire! Mix them into a salad or eat them by themselves, as you choose. Unlike fruit, you can enjoy a mixture of different vegetables on this Stage. (**Fresh Only!!!—Not frozen or canned or dried or juiced or cooked or micro-waved.**)
      You may put on lemon juice or any kind of vinegar.
      (**No Oil and No Salad Dressing.**) No avocado. No olives.

3.   At **one** meal per day all the **Lean, One Kind of Protein** you want to eat from the list below. (**Broiled or BBQ'd, No Sauces, No Bones, No Fat, No Skin.**)

Fish	No Shellfish
Beef	
	No chopped meat
	No ground meat
Veal	
Chicken	White Meat Only
Turkey	White Meat Only
Tuna	White Meat—Water Packed—Low Salt

<u>Sample Menu</u>
Cleansing & Relearning—Phase I
Stage A

Breakfast

Fruit of Day

Beverage (½ hour before meal, or ½ hour after meal)

Mid-Morning Snack

Fruit of Day

Beverage (½ hour before meal, or ½ hour after meal)

Lunch

Salad

Fruit of Day

Beverage (½ hour before meal, or ½ hour after meal)

Mid-Afternoon Snack

Fruit of Day

Beverage (½ hour before meal, or ½ hour after meal)

Dinner

Fruit of Day

Salad

Meat, Chicken, or Fish

Fruit of Day

Beverage (½ hour before meal, or ½ hour after meal)

Evening Snack

Fruit of Day

Diet Tips
Cleansing & Relearning—Phase I
Stage A

1. The most filling fruit is a grapefruit. An orange is the next most filling. After that come the melons.

2. If you are not getting filled up with the fruit you are eating, then spend more days eating the fruits listed above in Tip 1.

3. A good way to give the filet of chicken flavor is to marinate the chicken in vinegar, water, mustard, white horseradish, onion, and garlic, and then broil or BBQ.

4. It is O.K. to sprinkle Sweet 'n Low on grapefruit, strawberries or other fruit.

THE 18% SOLUTION
Cleansing & Relearning—Phase I
Stage B

1. All the **Fresh Fruit** you want to eat—you can mix fruit. (**Fresh Only!!!—Not frozen or canned or dried or juiced or cooked.**) No nuts. No seeds. No cocoanut. No watermelon. No grapes. No bananas.

2. All the **Fresh Raw Vegetables** you want to eat. You can have all the different kind of vegetables you desire! Mix them into a salad or eat them by themselves, as you choose. (**Fresh Only!!!—Not frozen or canned or dried or juiced or cooked or micro-waved.**) You may put on lemon juice or any kind of vinegar.
    (**No Oil and No Salad Dressing.**) No avocado. No olives.

3. At **one** meal per day all the **Lean, One Kind of Protein** you want to eat from the list below. (**Broiled or BBQ'd, No Sauces, No Bones, No Fat, No Skin.**)

Fish	No Shellfish
Beef	
	No chopped meat
	No ground meat
Veal	
Chicken	White Meat Only
Turkey	White Meat Only
Tuna	White Meat—Water Packed—Low Salt

<u>Sample Menu</u>
Cleansing & Relearning—Phase I
Stage B

Breakfast

Fruit

Beverage (½ hour before meal, or ½ hour after meal)

Mid-Morning Snack

Fruit

Beverage (½ hour before meal, or ½ hour after meal)

Lunch

Salad

Fruit

Beverage (½ hour before meal, or ½ hour after meal)

Mid-Afternoon Snack

Fruit

Beverage (½ hour before meal, or ½ hour after meal)

Dinner

Fruit

Salad

Meat, Chicken, or Fish

Fruit

Beverage (½ hour before meal, or ½ hour after meal)

Evening Snack

Fruit

<u>Diet Tips</u>
Cleansing & Relearning—Phase I
Stage B

1. **A good way not to get hungry** is to have some grapefruit each day.

2. It is O.K. to sprinkle Sweet 'n Low on grapefruit, strawberries or other fruit.

3. Eat some fruit at least 6 times per day, as designated in the sample menu, to keep from getting hungry, tired or weak.

THE 18% SOLUTION
Controlled, Healthy Weight Loss—Phase II
Stage C

1. All the **Fresh Fruit** you want to eat. You can mix fruit during this Stage. (**Fresh Only!!!—Not frozen or canned or dried or juiced or cooked.**) No nuts. No seeds. No cocoanut. No watermelon. No grapes. No bananas.

2. All the **Fresh Raw Vegetables** you want to eat. (**Fresh Only!!!—Not frozen or canned or dried or juiced or cooked or micro-waved.**) You can have all of the different kind of vegetables you desire! Mix them into a salad or eat them by themselves, as you choose. You may put on lemon juice or any kind of vinegar. (**No Oil and No Salad Dressing.**) No avocado. No olives.

3. At **one** meal per day all the **Lean, One Kind of Protein** you want to eat from the list below. (**Broiled or BBQ'd, No Sauces, No Bones, No Fat, No Skin.**)

Fish	No Shellfish
Beef	
	No chopped meat
	No ground meat
Veal	
Chicken	White Meat Only
Turkey	White Meat Only
Tuna	White Meat—Water Packed—Low Salt

All of the following items in the rest of this section (after item 3 above) are permissible up to four times a week, since they are considered treats:

4. At **one meal** per day other than the main meal, you have one of the following:

    4 oz. Non-Fat Cottage Cheese

    4 oz. Non-Fat Unflavored, Plain Yogurt

    8 oz. Non-Fat Milk

    4 oz. Non-Fat Frozen Yogurt—Sugar Free

    2 Egg Whites—No Yolks

    4 oz. Tuna—White Meat—Water Packed—Low Salt

<u>Sample Menu</u>
Controlled, Healthy Weight Loss—Phase II
Stage C

Breakfast

Fruit

Beverage (½ hour before meal, ½ hour after meal)

Mid-Morning Snack

Fruit

Beverage (½ hour before meal, or ½ hour after meal)

Lunch

Salad

Fruit

Non-Fat Cottage Cheese, Yogurt, or White Meat Water Packed Tuna

Beverage (½ hour before meal, or ½ hour after meal)

Mid-Afternoon Snack

Fruit

Beverage (½ hour before meal, ½ hour after meal)

Dinner

Fruit

Salad

Meat, Chicken, or Fish

Fruit

Beverage (½ hour before meal, or ½ hour after meal)

Evening Snack

Fruit

Diet Tips
Controlled, Healthy Weight Loss—Phase II
Stage C

1. You must pour out the liquid from the water packed tuna. Then rinse the tuna under water 3 times to wash away the high salt content. It must be low salt tuna.

2. Cut fruit such as strawberries, peaches or raspberries into your yogurt and cottage cheese.

3. You may add lemon juice and Sweet 'n Low to the yogurt or cottage cheese.

4. Make an egg white omelet by using the white of the egg, adding pepper, onion, garlic, vegetables and beating with a fork. Put into microwave safe bowel and cook at high power for 60 seconds per egg or to the consistency you like.

THE 18% SOLUTION
Controlled, Healthy Weight Loss—Phase II
Stage D

1. All of the **Fresh Fruit you want to eat—you can mix fruit**. (**Fresh Only!!!—Not frozen or canned or dried or juiced or cooked**.) No nuts. No seeds. No cocoanut. No watermelon. No grapes. No bananas.

2. All the **Fresh Raw Vegetables** you want to eat. (**Fresh Only!!!—Not frozen or canned or dried or juiced or cooked or micro-waved**.) You can have all of the different kind of vegetables you desire! Mix them into a salad or eat them by themselves, as you choose. You may put on lemon juice or any kind of vinegar.
    (**No Oil and No Salad Dressing**.) No avocado. No olives.

3. At **one** meal per day you can have all the **Lean, One Kind of Protein** you want to eat from the list below. (**Broiled or BBQ'd, No Sauces, No Bones, No Fat, No Skin**.)

Fish	No Shellfish
Beef	
	No chopped meat
	No ground meat
Veal	
Chicken	White Meat Only
Turkey	White Meat Only
Tuna	White Meat—Water Packed—Low Salt

All of the following items in the rest of this section (after item 3 above) are permissible up to four times a week, since they are considered treats:

4.   At **two meals** per day other than the main meal, you have one of the following:

   4 oz. Non-Fat Cottage Cheese

   4 oz. Non-Fat Unflavored, Plain Yogurt

   8 oz. Non-Fat Milk

   4 oz. Non-Fat Frozen Yogurt—Sugar Free

   2 Egg Whites—No Yolks

   4 oz. Tuna—White Meat—Water Packed—Low Salt

Sample Menu
Controlled, Healthy Weight Loss—Phase II
Stage D

Breakfast

Fruit

Non-Fat Cottage Cheese, Yogurt, or Milk

Beverage (½ hour before meal, or ½ hour after meal)

Mid-Morning Snack

Fruit

Beverage (½ hour before meal, ½ after meal)

Lunch

Salad

Fruit

Non-Fat Cottage Cheese, Yogurt, or White Meat Water Packed Tuna

Beverage (½ hour before meal, or ½ after meal)

Mid-Afternoon Snack

Fruit

Beverage (½ hour before meal, ½ hour after meal)

Dinner

Fruit

Salad

Meat, Chicken or Fish

Beverage (½ hour before meal, ½ hour after meal)

Evening Snack

Fruit

Diet Tips
Controlled, Healthy Weight Loss—Phase II
Stage D

1. Although you can eat a protein for breakfast and lunch, you do not have to. Eat a protein only the days you want to.

2. You can eat the same protein for breakfast and lunch, or vary them if you want to.

THE 18% SOLUTION
Maintenance Phase—Phase III
Stage E

1. All the **Fresh Fruit you want to eat—you can mix fruit**. (**Fresh Only!!!—Not frozen or canned or dried or juiced or cooked.**) No nuts. No seeds. No cocoanut. No watermelon. No grapes. No bananas.

2. All the **Fresh Raw Vegetables** you want to eat. You can have all of the different kind of vegetables you desire! Mix them into a salad or eat them by themselves, as you choose. (**Fresh Only!!!—Not frozen or canned or dried or juiced or cooked or micro-waved.**) You may put on lemon juice or any kind of vinegar.
    (**No Oil and No Salad Dressing.**) No avocado. No olives.

3. At **one** meal per day you can have all the **Lean, One Kind of Protein** you want to eat from the list below. (**Broiled or BBQ'd, No Sauces, No Bones, No Fat, No Skin.**)

Fish	No Shellfish
Beef	
	No chopped meat
	No ground meat
Veal	
Chicken	White Meat Only
Turkey	White Meat Only
Tuna	White Meat—Water Packed—Low Salt

All of the following items in the rest of this section (after item 3 above) are permissible up to four times a week, since they are considered treats:

4. At **two meals** per day other than the main meal, you can have one of the following:

    4 oz. Non-Fat Cottage Cheese

    4 oz. Non-Fat Unflavored, Plain Yogurt

    8 oz. Non-Fat Milk

    4 oz. Non-Fat Frozen Yogurt—Sugar Free

    2 Egg Whites—No Yolks

    4 oz. Tuna—White Meat—Water Packed—Low Salt

5. At **one meal** per day you can have only one of the following starches:

    1 Baked Potato—Whole Only—plain, no dressing

    1 Baked Yam—Whole Only

    1 Corn on the Cob—Whole Only—Fresh Only

<u>Sample Menu</u>
Maintenance Phase—Phase III
Stage E

Breakfast

> Fruit
>
> Non-Fat Cottage Cheese, Yogurt, or Milk
>
> Beverage (½ hour before meal, or ½ hour after meal)

Mid-Morning Snack

> Fruit
>
> Beverage (½ hour before meal, or ½ hour after meal)

Lunch

> Salad
>
> Fruit
>
> Non-Fat Cottage Cheese, Yogurt, or White Meat Water Packed Tuna
>
> Beverage (½ hour before meal, or ½ hour after meal)

Mid-Afternoon Snack

> Fruit
>
> Beverage (½ hour before meal, or ½ hour after meal)

Dinner

> Fruit
>
> Salad
>
> Meat, Chicken, or Fish
>
> **Baked Potato, Yam, or Corn on the Cob**
>
> Fruit
>
> Beverage (½ hour before meal, or ½ hour after meal)

Evening Snack

> Fruit

<u>Diet Tips</u>
Maintenance Phase—Phase III
Stage E

1. You can put mustard or vinegar or a combination on the potato or corn to give it flavor.

2. You do not need to eat a potato or corn every day. Eat them only when you feel like it.

3. You do not have to eat a big potato, or eat the entire potato. Take as much as you want up to one whole potato.

4. It is best not to have starches every day.

THE 18% SOLUTION
Maintenance Phase—Phase III
Stage F

1. All of the **Fresh Fruit you want to eat—you can mix fruit**. (**Fresh Only!!!—Not frozen or canned or dried or juiced or cooked.**) No nuts. No seeds. No cocoanut. No watermelon. No grapes. No bananas.

2. All the **Fresh Raw Vegetables** you want to eat. You can have all of the different kind of vegetables you desire! Mix them into a salad or eat them by themselves, as you choose. (**Fresh Only!!!—Not frozen or canned or dried or juiced or cooked or micro-waved.**) You may put on lemon juice or any kind of vinegar.
    (**No Oil and No Salad Dressing.**) No avocado. No olives.

3. At **one** meal per day you can have all the **Lean, One Kind of Protein** you want to eat from the list below. (**Broiled or BBQ'd, No Sauces, No Bones, No Fat, No Skin.**)

Fish	No Shellfish
Beef	
	No chopped meat
	No ground meat
Veal	
Chicken	White Meat Only
Turkey	White Meat Only
Tuna	White Meat—Water Packed—Low Salt

All of the following items in the rest of this section (after item 3 above) are permissible up to four times a week, since they are considered treats:

4.   At **two meals** other than the main meal per day, you have one of the following:

4 oz. Non-Fat Cottage Cheese

4 oz. Non-Fat Unflavored, Plain Yogurt

8 oz. Non-Fat Milk

4 oz. Non-Fat Frozen Yogurt—Sugar Free

2 Egg Whites—No Yolks

4 oz. Tuna—White Meat—Water Packed—Low Salt

5.   At **one meal** per day you can have only one of the following starches:

1 Baked Potato—Whole Only—plain, no dressing

1 Baked Yam—Whole Only

1 Corn on the Cob—Whole Only—Fresh Only

6.   At breakfast you can have **one** from the following:

1 Slice of Bread (pre-sliced by bakery) Fresh or Toasted

1 Portion—¾ cup, dry unsweetened cereal which has no fat, e.g., Cornflakes

Sample Menu
Maintenance Phase—Phase III
Stage F

Breakfast

Fruit

Bread or Cereal

Non-Fat Cottage Cheese, Yogurt, or Milk

Beverage (½ hour before meal, or ½ hour after meal)

Mid-Morning Snack

Fruit

Beverage (½ hour before meal, or ½ hour after meal)

Lunch

Salad

Fruit

Non-Fat Cottage Cheese, Yogurt, or White Meat Water Packed Tuna

Beverage (½ hour before meal, or ½ hour after meal)

Mid-Afternoon Snack

Fruit

Beverage (½ hour before meal, or ½ hour after meal)

Dinner

Fruit

Salad

Meat, Chicken, Veal or Fish

Baked Potato, Yam, or Corn on the Cob

Fruit

Beverage (½ hour before meal, or ½ hour after meal)

Evening Snack

Fruit

Diet Tips
Maintenance Phase—Phase III
Stage F

1. If you have cereal, you should choose the Non-Fat Milk as your protein for breakfast so that you have milk for the cereal.

2. You do not have to have bread or cereal every day. Choose it only when you want to.

3. You do not have to have a whole slice of bread, or the whole ¾ cup of cereal.

4. You may want to put cottage cheese on your bread.

5. You may want to put mustard or horseradish on your bread.

6. You may want to add fruit to your cereal.

7. It is best not to eat starches every day.

THE 18% SOLUTION
Maintenance Phase—Phase III
Stage G

1. All of the **Fresh Fruit you want to eat—you can mix fruit**. (**Fresh Only!!!—Not frozen or canned or dried or juiced or cooked**.) No nuts. No seeds. No cocoanut. No watermelon. No grapes. No bananas.

2. All the **Fresh Raw Vegetables** you want to eat. You can have all of the different kind of vegetables you desire! Mix them into a salad or eat them by themselves, as you choose. (**Fresh Only!!!—Not frozen or canned or dried or juiced or cooked or micro-waved**.) You may put on lemon juice or any kind of vinegar.
    (**No Oil and No Salad Dressing**.) No avocado. No olives.

3. At **one** meal per day you can have all the **Lean, One Kind of Protein** you want to eat from the list below. (**Broiled or BBQ'd, No Sauces, No Bones, No Fat, No Skin**.)

Fish	No Shellfish
Beef	
	No chopped meat
	No ground meat
Veal	
Chicken	White Meat Only
Turkey	White Meat Only
Tuna	White Meat—Water Packed—Low Salt

All of the following items in the rest of this section (after item 3 above) are permissible up to four times a week, since they are considered treats:

4. At **two meals** other than the main meal per day, you can have one of the following:

    4 oz. Non-Fat Cottage Cheese

    4 oz. Non-Fat Unflavored, Plain Yogurt

    8 oz. Non-Fat Milk

    4 oz. Non-Fat Frozen Yogurt—Sugar Free

    2 Egg Whites—No Yolks

    4 oz. Tuna—White Meat—Water Packed—Low Salt

5. At **one meal** per day you can have only one of the following starches:

    1 Baked Potato—Whole Only—plain, no dressing

    1 Baked Yam—Whole Only

    1 Corn on the Cob—Whole Only—Fresh Only

    ½ Cup—(after cooked) Rice—cooked in water only

    No Sauces—Not Fried—Not Sautéed

6. At breakfast you can have **one** from the following:

    1 Slice of Bread (pre-sliced by bakery) Fresh or Toasted

    1 Portion—¾ cup, dry unsweetened cereal which has no fat, e.g., Corn-flakes

<u>Sample Menu</u>
Maintenance Phase—Phase III
Stage G

Breakfast

Fruit

Bread or Cereal

Non-Fat Cottage Cheese, or Milk

Beverage (½ hour before meal, or ½ hour after meal)

Mid-Morning Snack

Fruit

Beverage (½ hour before meal, or ½ hour after meal)

Lunch

Salad

Fruit

Non-Fat Cottage Cheese, Yogurt, or White Meat Water Packed Tuna

Mid-Afternoon Snack

Fruit

Beverage (½ hour before meal, or ½ hour after meal)

Dinner

Fruit

Salad

Meat, Chicken, or Fish

Baked Potato, Yam, Corn on the Cob or **Rice**

Fruit

Beverage (½ hour before meal, or ½ hour after meal)

Evening Snack

Fruit

Diet Tips
Maintenance Phase—Phase III
Stage G

1. Rice must be cooked only in water, no salt or oil or margarine.

2. You must be careful not to eat more than **½ cup of cooked rice.**

3. You do not need to eat even the whole ½ cup of cooked rice.

4. Eat the rice only if you want to.

5. It is best not to eat starches every day.

THE 18% SOLUTION
Maintenance Phase—Phase III
Stage H

1.   All of the **Fresh Fruit you want to eat—you can mix fruit**. (**Fresh Only!!!—Not frozen or canned or dried or juiced or cooked.**) No nuts. No seeds. No cocoanut. No watermelon. No grapes. No bananas.

2.   All the **Fresh Raw Vegetables** you want to eat. (**Fresh Only!!!—Not frozen or canned or dried or juiced or cooked or micro-waved.**) You can have all of the different kind of vegetables you desire! Mix them into a salad or eat them by themselves, as you choose. You may put on lemon juice or any kind of vinegar.
      (**No Oil and No Salad Dressing.**) No avocado. No olives.

3.   At **one** meal per day you can have all the **Lean, One Kind of Protein** you want to eat from the list below. (**Broiled or BBQ'd, No Sauces, No Bones, No Fat, No Skin.**)

Fish	No Shellfish
Beef	
	No chopped meat
	No ground meat
Veal	
Chicken	White Meat Only
Turkey	White Meat Only
Tuna	White Meat—Water Packed—Low Salt

All of the following items in the rest of this section (after item 3 above) are permissible up to four times a week, since they are considered treats:

4.   At **two meals** other than the main meal per day, you can have one of the following:

   4 oz. Non-Fat Cottage Cheese

   4 oz. Non-Fat Unflavored, Plain Yogurt

   8 oz. Non-Fat Milk

   4 oz. Non-Fat Frozen Yogurt—Sugar Free

   2 Egg Whites—No Yolks

   4 oz. Tuna—White Meat—Water Packed—Low Salt

5.   At **one meal** per day you can have only one of the following starches:

   1 Baked Potato—Whole Only—plain, no dressing

   1 Baked Yam—Whole Only

   1 Corn on the Cob—Whole Only—Fresh Only

   ½ Cup—(after cooked) Rice—cooked in water only

   No Sauces—Not Fried—Not Sautéed

6.   At breakfast you can have **one** from the following:

   1 Slice of Bread (pre-sliced by bakery) Fresh or Toasted

   1 Portion—¾ cup, dry unsweetened cereal which has no fat, e.g., Cornflakes

7.   At **one meal** per day you can have 1 cup of steamed or barbecued vegetables. **This does not include potatoes or corn as a vegetable.**

Sample Menu
Maintenance Phase—Phase III
Stage H

Breakfast

> Fruit
>
> Bread or Cereal
>
> Non-Fat Cottage Cheese, Yogurt, or Milk
>
> Beverage (½ hour before meal, or ½ hour after meal)

Mid-Morning Snack

> Fruit
>
> Beverage (½ hour before meal, or ½ hour after meal)

Lunch

> Salad
>
> Fruit
>
> Non-Fat Cottage Cheese, Yogurt, or White Meat Water Packed Tuna
>
> Beverage (½ hour before meal, or ½ hour after meal)

Mid-Afternoon Snack

> Fruit
>
> Beverage (½ hour before meal, or ½ hour after meal)

Dinner

> Fruit
>
> Salad
>
> Meat, Chicken, or Fish
>
> Baked Potato, Yam, Corn on the Cob or Rice
>
> **Steamed, Broiled or BBQ'd Green Vegetables**
>
> Fruit
>
> Beverage (½ hour before meal, or ½ hour after meal)

Evening Snack

> Fruit

Diet Tips
Maintenance Phase—Phase III
Stage H

1. You can have only up to 1 cup of steamed or barbecued vegetables. **This does not include potatoes or corn as a vegetable.**

2. You do not need to have steamed vegetables every day.

3. It is best not to have steamed vegetables every day. Eat them only on the days you really want them.

4. The vegetables **cannot** be cooked in salt or with margarine or oil.

5. The vegetables for best taste should be barbecued or broiled.

6. The vegetables must not be cooked long. They must be relatively hard when finished.

THE 18% SOLUTION
Maintenance Phase—Phase III
Stage I

1. All of the **Fresh Fruit you want to eat—you can mix fruit**. (**Fresh Only!!!—Not frozen or canned or dried or juiced or cooked.**) No nuts. No seeds. No cocoanut. No watermelon. No grapes. No bananas.

2. All the **Fresh Raw Vegetables** you want to eat. You can have all of the different kind of vegetables you desire! Mix them into a salad or eat them by themselves, as you choose. (**Fresh Only!!!—Not Frozen or canned or dried or juiced or cooked or micro-waved.**) You may put on lemon juice or any kind of vinegar.
    (**No Oil and No Salad dressing.**) No avocado. No olives.

3. At **one** meal per day you can have all the **Lean, One Kind of Protein** you want to eat from the list below. (**Broiled or BBQ'd, No Sauces, No Bones, No Fat, No Skin.**)

Fish	No Shellfish
Beef	
	No chopped meat
	No ground meat
Veal	
Chicken	White Meat Only
Turkey	White Meat Only
Tuna	White Meat—Water Packed—Low Salt

<u>All of the following items in the rest of this section (after item 3</u>
<u>above) are permissible up to four times a week, since they are</u>
<u>considered treats:</u>

4.   At **two meals** other than the main meal per day, you can have one of the
     following:

     4 oz. Non-Fat Cottage Cheese

     4 oz. Non-Fat Unflavored, Plain Yogurt

     8 oz. Non-Fat Milk

     4 oz. Non-Fat Frozen Yogurt—Sugar Free

     2 Egg Whites—No Yolks

     4 oz. Tuna—White Meat—Water Packed—Low Salt

5.   At **one meal** per day you can have only one of the following starches:

     1 Baked Potato—Whole Only—plain, no dressing

     1 Baked Yam—Whole Only

     1 Corn on the Cob—Whole Only—Fresh Only

     ½ Cup—(after cooked) Rice—cooked in water only

     <u>No Sauces—Not Fried—Not Sautéed</u>

6.   At breakfast you can have **one** from the following:

     1 Slice of Bread (pre-sliced by bakery) Fresh or Toasted

     1 Portion—¾ cup, dry unsweetened cereal which has no fat, e.g., Corn-
     flakes

7.   You can have only up to 1 cup of steamed or barbecued vegetables. **This**
     does not include potatoes or corn as a vegetable.

8.   At **one meal** per day you can have a bowl of homemade vegetable soup.
     Make from fresh vegetables. **Do not include starches, oil, margarine,**
     meat, or bones.

<u>Sample Menu</u>
Maintenance Phase—Phase III
Stage I

Breakfast

Fruit

Bread or cereal

Non-Fat Cottage Cheese, Yogurt, or Milk

Beverage (½ hour before meal, or ½ hour after meal)

Mid-Morning Snack

Fruit

Beverage (½ hour before meal, or ½ hour after meal)

Lunch

Salad

Fruit

Non-Fat Cottage Cheese, Yogurt, or White Meat Water Packed Tuna

Beverage (½ hour before meal, or ½ hour after meal)

Mid-Afternoon Snack

Fruit

Beverage (½ hour before meal, or ½ hour after meal)

Dinner

Fruit

Homemade Vegetable Soup

Salad

Meat, Chicken, or Fish

Baked Potato, Yam, Corn on the Cob or Rice

Steamed, Broiled or BBQ vegetables

Fruit

Beverage (½ hour before meal, or ½ hour after meal)

Evening Snack

Fruit

<u>Diet Tips</u>
Maintenance Phase—Phase III
Stage I

1.   The soup must be homemade.

2.   You can have up to 8 oz. of soup per day. You do not have to eat that much.

3.   It is best not to have the soup every day. Eat it only when you really want some soup.

4.   There can be no oil, margarine, salt, bones or meat in the soup.

5.   It tastes better if you use broiled or barbecued vegetables in the soup.

6.   You may put the soup through a blender.

THE 18% SOLUTION
Maintenance Phase—Phase III
Stage J

1. All of the **Fresh Fruit you want to eat—you can mix fruit. (Fresh Only!!!—Not frozen or canned or dried or juiced or cooked.)** No nuts. No seeds. No cocoanut. No watermelon. No grapes. No bananas.

2. All the **Fresh Raw Vegetables** you want to eat. You can have all of the different kind of vegetables you desire! Mix them into a salad or eat them by themselves, as you choose. (**Fresh Only!!!—Not frozen or canned or dried or juiced or cooked or micro-waved.**) You may put on lemon juice or any kind of vinegar.
(**No Oil and No Salad Dressing.**) No avocado. No olives.

3. At **one** meal per day you can have all the **Lean, One Kind of Protein** you want to eat from the list below. (**Broiled or BBQ'd, No Sauces, No Bones, No Fat, No Skin.**)

Fish	No Shellfish
Beef	
	No chopped meat
	No ground meat
Veal	
Chicken	White Meat Only
Turkey	White Meat Only
Tuna	White Meat—Water Packed—Low Salt

<u>All of the following items in the rest of this section (after item 3</u>
<u>above) are permissible up to four times a week, since they are</u>
<u>considered treats:</u>

4.   At **two meals** other than the main meal per day, you can have one of the
      following:

      4 oz. Non-Fat Cottage Cheese

      4 oz. Non-Fat Unflavored, Plain Yogurt

      8 oz. Non-Fat Milk

      4 oz. Non-Fat Frozen Yogurt—Sugar Free

      2 Egg Whites—No Yolks

      4 oz. Tuna—White Meat—Water Packed—Low Salt

5.   At **one meal** per day you can have only **one** of the following starches:

      1 Baked Potato—Whole Only—plain, no dressing

      1 Baked Yam—Whole Only

      1 Corn on the Cob—Whole Only—Fresh Only

      ½ Cup—(after cooked) Rice—cooked in water only—
            No Sauces

      ½ Cup—(after cooked) Pasta—cooked in water only—
            No Sauces

      <u>No Sauces—Not Fried—Not Sautéed</u>

6.   At breakfast you can have **one** from the following:

      1 Slice of Bread (pre-sliced by bakery) Fresh or Toasted

      1 Portion—¾ cup, dry unsweetened cereal which has no fat, e.g., Corn-
      flakes

7.   You can have only up to 1 cup of steamed or barbecued vegetables. **This**
      does not include potatoes or corn as a vegetable.

8.   At **one meal** per day you can have a bowl of homemade vegetable soup.
      Make from fresh vegetables. **Do not include starches, oil, margarine,**
      meat, or bones.

Sample Menu
Maintenance Phase—Phase III
Stage J

Breakfast

Fruit

Bread or Cereal

Non-Fat Cottage Cheese, Yogurt, or Milk

Beverage (½ hour before meal, or ½ hour after meal)

Mid-Morning Snack

Fruit

Beverage (½ hour before meal, or ½ hour after meal)

Lunch

Salad

Fruit

Non-Fat Cottage Cheese, Yogurt, or White Meat Water Packed Tuna

Beverage (½ hour before meal, or ½ hour after meal)

Mid-Afternoon Snack

Fruit

Beverage (½ hour before meal, or ½ hour after meal)

Dinner

Fruit

Homemade Vegetable Soup

Salad

Meat, Chicken, or Fish

Baked Potato, Yam, Corn on the Cob, Rice or **Pasta**

Steamed, Broiled or BBQ'd Green Vegetables

Fruit

Beverage (½ hour before meal, or ½ hour after meal)

Evening Snack

Fruit

Diet Tips
Maintenance Phase—Phase III
Stage J

1. You may have only up to a ½ cup of pasta after it is cooked.

2. The pasta can be cooked in water only. You may not use oil, margarine or salt.

3. You do not have to eat a full ½ cup of cooked pasta. Eat as much as you want up to the ½ cup.

4. It is best not to have starch every day.

5. You may not cook it in any sauces.

6. You must cook the pasta yourself.

7. You can make a sauce yourself, with fresh raw vegetables and vinegar and herbs.

THE 18% SOLUTION
Maintenance Phase—Phase III
Stage K

1.   All of the **Fresh Fruit you want to eat—you can mix fruit**. (**Fresh Only!!!—Not frozen or canned or dried or juiced or cooked.**) No nuts. No seeds. No cocoanut. No watermelon. No grapes. No bananas.

2.   All the **Fresh Raw Vegetables** you want to eat. You can have all of the different kind of vegetables you desire! Mix them into a salad or eat them by themselves, as you choose. (**Fresh Only!!!—Not Frozen or canned or dried or juiced or cooked or micro-waved.**) You may put on lemon juice or any kind of vinegar.
      (**No Oil and No Salad dressing.**) No avocado. No olives.

3.   At **one** meal per day you can have all the **Lean, One Kind of Protein** you want to eat from the list below. (**Broiled or BBQ'd, No Sauces, No Bones, No Fat, No Skin.**)

Fish	No Shellfish
Beef	
	No chopped meat
	No ground meat
Veal	
Chicken	White Meat Only
Turkey	White Meat Only
Tuna	White Meat—Water Packed—Low Salt

All of the following items in the rest of this section (after item 3 above) are permissible up to four times a week, since they are considered treats:

4. At **two meals** other than the main meal per day, you can have one of the following:

   4 oz. Non-Fat Cottage Cheese

   4 oz. Non-Fat Unflavored, Plain Yogurt

   8 oz. Non-Fat Milk

   4 oz. Non-Fat Frozen Yogurt—Sugar Free

   2 Egg Whites—No Yolks

   4 oz. Tuna—White Meat—Water Packed—Low Salt

5. At **one meal** per day you can have only one of the following starches:

   1 Baked Potato—Whole Only—plain, no dressing

   1 Baked Yam—Whole Only

   1 Corn on the Cob—Whole Only—Fresh Only

   ½ Cup—(after cooked) Rice—cooked in water only—

   　　No Sauces

   ½ Cup—(after cooked) Pasta—cooked in water only—

   　　No Sauces

   No Sauces—Not Fried—Not Sautéed

6. At breakfast you can have **one** from the following:

   1 Slice of Bread (pre-sliced by bakery) Fresh or Toasted

   1 Portion—¾ cup, dry unsweetened cereal which has no fat, e.g., Corn-flakes

7. You can have only up to 1 cup of steamed or barbecued vegetables. **This does not include potatoes or corn as a vegetable.**

8.   At **one meal** per day you can have a bowl of homemade vegetable soup. Make from fresh vegetables. **Do not include starches, oil, margarine, meat, or bones.**

9.   Up to 2 times per week (not on the same day), you can have 4 oz. **dry white or red wine** with dinner.

Sample Menu
Maintenance Phase—Phase III
Stage K

Breakfast

Fruit

Bread or Cereal

Non-Fat Cottage Cheese, Yogurt, or Milk

Beverage (½ hour before meal, or ½ hour after meal)

Mid-Morning Snack

Fruit

Beverage (½ hour before meal, or ½ hour after meal)

Lunch

Salad

Fruit

Non-Fat Cottage Cheese, Yogurt, or White Meat Water Packed Tuna

Beverage (½ hour before meal, or ½ hour after meal)

Mid-Afternoon Snack

Fruit

Beverage (½ hour before meal, or ½ hour after meal)

Dinner

Fruit

Homemade Vegetable Soup

Salad

Meat, Chicken, or Fish

Baked Potato, Yam, Corn on the Cob, Rice or Pasta

Steamed, Broiled or BBQ'd Vegetables

Fruit

Beverage (½ hour before meal, or ½ after meal)

4 oz. white or red dry wine

Evening Snack

Fruit

Diet Tips
Maintenance Phase—Phase III
Stage K

1. You msy drink the wine, a little before or after the meal. (You do not have to wait a full 30 minutes.)

2. You cannot have the 2 glasses of wine in one day.

3. It must be dry wine, not semi-dry or sweet wine.

4. No liquor.

5. No beer.

THE 18% SOLUTION
Maintenance Phase—Phase III
Stage L

1. All of the **Fresh Fruit you want to eat—you can mix fruit**. (**Fresh Only!!!—Not frozen or canned or dried or juiced or cooked.**) No nuts. No seeds. No cocoanut. No watermelon. No grapes. No bananas.

2. All the **Fresh Raw Vegetables** you want to eat. You can have all of the different kind of vegetables you desire! Mix them into a salad or eat them by themselves, as you choose. (**Fresh Only!!!—Not Frozen or canned or dried or juiced or cooked or micro-waved.**) You may put on lemon juice or any kind of vinegar. (**No Oil and No Salad dressing.**) No avocado. No olives.

3. At **one** meal per day you can have all the **Lean, One Kind of Protein** you want to eat from the list below. (**Broiled or BBQ'd, No Sauces, No Bones, No Fat, No Skin.**)

Fish	No Shellfish
Beef	
	No chopped meat
	No ground meat
Veal	
Chicken	White Meat Only
Turkey	White Meat Only
Tuna	White Meat—Water Packed—Low Salt

All of the following items in the rest of this section (after item 3 above) are permissible up to four times a week, since they are considered treats:

4. At **two meals** other than the main meal per day, you can have one of the following:

    4 oz. Non-Fat Cottage Cheese

    4 oz. Non-Fat Unflavored, Plain Yogurt

    8 oz. Non-Fat Milk

    4 oz. Non-Fat Frozen Yogurt—Sugar Free

    2 Egg Whites—No Yolks

    4 oz. Tuna—White Meat—Water Packed—Low Salt

5. At **one meal** per day you can have only one of the following starches:

    1 Baked Potato—Whole Only—plain, no dressing

    1 Baked Yam—Whole Only

    1 Corn on the Cob—Whole Only—Fresh Only

    ½ Cup—(after cooked) Rice—cooked in water only—

    No Sauces

    ½ Cup—(after cooked) Pasta—cooked in water only—

    No Sauces

    No Sauces—Not Fried—Not Sautéed

6. At breakfast you can have **one** from the following:

    1 Slice of Bread (pre-sliced by bakery) Fresh or Toasted

    1 Portion—¾ cup, dry unsweetened cereal which has no fat, e.g., Cornflakes

7. You can have only up to 1 cup of steamed or barbecued vegetables. **This does not include potatoes or corn as a vegetable.**

8. At **one meal** per day you can have a bowl of homemade vegetable soup. Make from fresh vegetables. **Do not include starches, oil, margarine, meat, or bones.**

9. Up to 2 times per week (not on the same day) you can have 4 oz. dry white or red wine with dinner.

10. Up to 4 times per week, for a snack you can have up to 2 cups (when completed) air-popped, plain popcorn.

Sample Menu
Maintenance Phase—Phase III
Stage L

Breakfast

Fruit

Bread or Cereal

Non-Fat Cottage Cheese, Yogurt or Milk

Beverage

Mid-Morning Snack

Fruit

Beverage

Lunch

Salad

Fruit

Non-Fat Cottage Cheese, Yogurt or White Meat Water Packed Tuna

Beverage

Mid-Afternoon Snack

Fruit

Beverage

Dinner

Fruit

Homemade Vegetable Soup

Salad

Meat, Chicken, or Fish

Baked Potato, Yam, Corn on the Cob, Rice or Pasta

Steamed Broiled or BBQ'd Vegetables

Fruit

Beverage

4 oz. white or red dry wine

Evening Snack

Fruit

2 Cups Air-Popped Popcorn

Diet Tips
Maintenance Phase—Phase III
Stage L

1. You must start with whole kernels and air pop or microwave.

2. No more than 2 cups after popped.

3. You may not have commercially popped popcorn at the movies or from package.

4. No toppings such as salt or butter.

THE 18% SOLUTION
Cleansing & Relearning—Phase I
Stage X

1. All of the **Fresh Fruit you want to eat—you can mix fruit.** You may change your selection each day. (**Fresh Only!!!—Not frozen or canned or dried or juiced or cooked**). No Nuts. No Seeds. No Coconut. No Watermelon. No Grapes. No Bananas.

2. All the **Fresh Raw Vegetables** you want to eat. You can have all of the different kind of vegetables you desire! Mix them into a salad or eat them by themselves, as you choose. (**Fresh Only!!!—Not Frozen or canned or dried or juiced or cooked or micro-waved.**) You may put on lemon juice or any kind of vinegar.
    (**No Oil and No Salad dressing.**) No avocado. No olives.

3. Up to Six (**6**) hard boiled eggs per day.

<u>Sample Menu</u>
Cleansing & Relearning—Phase I
Stage X

Breakfast

Fruit

Beverage

1 Hard Boiled Egg

Mid-Morning Snack

Fruit

Beverage

Lunch

Salad

Fruit

Beverage

1 Hard Boiled Egg

Mid-Afternoon Snack

Fruit

Beverage

1 Hard Boiled Egg

Dinner

Fruit

Salad

3 Hard Boiled Eggs

Fruit

Beverage

Evening Snack

Fruit

<u>Diet Tips</u>
Cleansing & Relearning—Phase I
Stage X

1.   A good way not to get hungry is to have some grapefruit each day.

2.   It is O.K. to sprinkle sweet-n-low on grapefruit, strawberries or other fruit.

3.   Eat some fruit at least 6 times per day, as designated in the sample menu, to keep from getting hungry, tired or weak.

4.   Eggs may be eaten any time, a maximum of 6 whole hard boiled eggs per day.

THE 18% SOLUTION
Salad—Examples—All Stages

1. Iceberg lettuce, tomato, cucumbers, and carrots,

2. Zucchini slaw and apple with lemon juice

3. Tomatoes and onions and basil

4. Diced cumbers and diced tomatoes

5. Spinach and strawberries

6. Endives and tomatoes

7. Cabbage slaw and pineapples with lemon juice

8. Romaine lettuce with mushrooms, peppers and radishes

9. Arrugula and orange

10. Carrots and pineapple and lemon juice

11. Spinach and mango

12. Lettuce, onions, green pepper, and jicama

13. Raw cauliflower, and raw broccoli with Dijon mustard and vinegar dressing

14. Butter-lettuce, arrugula and romaine lettuce

THE 18% SOLUTION
Salad Dressings—Examples—All Stages

1. Vinegar (any kind individually or mixed, such as unseasoned rice, balsamic, wine, apple or grain.)

2. Vinegar, mustard (any kind such as plain, Dijon, honey or deli), water, garlic, pepper, onion powder, white horseradish, Splenda. (you can use all these ingredients or some of them.

3. Lemon juice

THE 18% SOLUTION
Main Dish—Examples—All Stages

1. Tenderloin steak and salad

2. Grilled chicken breast slices in a salad

3. Salmon steak in lettuce leaf with salad as a side

4. Grilled veal slices in a salad

5. Rib eye steak and salad

6. Grilled fillet of Red Snapper pieces in a salad

7. Grilled turkey breast in lettuce leaf with salad as a side

8. Tenderloin Steak pieces in a salad

9. Grilled veal in lettuce leaf with salad as a side

10. Grilled chicken breast and salad

11. Grilled fillet of flounder in lettuce leaf with salad as a side

(Continued)

12.   Fillet of sole pieces in a salad

13.   Grilled turkey breast and salad

14.   Tenderloin steak in lettuce leaf with salad as a side

15.   Salmon steak and salad

16.   Grilled fillet of veal and salad

17.   Grilled turkey breast pieces in a salad

18.   Minute steak in lettuce leaf with salad as a side

19.   Grilled fillet of halibut and salad

20.   Rib eye steak on a salad

21.   Grilled chicken breast in lettuce leaf with salad as a side

THE 18% SOLUTION
Secondary Meal—Examples—Stage C And Up

1. 4 oz. fat free cottage cheese and mixed fruit

2. 4 oz plain fat free yogurt and fresh berries (you must add the fruit)

3. 8 oz fat free milk and fruit

4. 12 oz decaffeinated latte coffee with fat free milk (no powders)

5. 4 oz white meat water packed—low salt tuna (no mayonnaise, not tuna salad) and mixed lettuce salad

6. 4 oz frozen yogurt—sugar free—and fat free (such as Carbolite) and fresh berries

7. 2 egg whites and tomatoes (Egg whites from fresh eggs not eggbeaters).

    a. hard boil the 2 eggs and through away the yoke

    b. poach the 2 egg whites in water with no salt

    c. scramble the 2 egg whites and microwave them

    d. scramble the 2 egg whites and cook them on a non stick skillet (you may not use Pam)

www.ingramcontent.com/pod-product-compliance
Lightning Source LLC
Chambersburg PA
CBHW051419280526
45785CB00003B/1086